Echocardiography Board Review

400 Multiple Choice Questions with Discussion

Ramdas G. Pai MD, FACC, FRCP (Edin)
Director of Integrated Cardiovascular Imaging Center
Loma Linda University Medical Center, Loma Linda, CA, USA

and

Padmini Varadarajan MD, FACC
Advanced Cardiovascular Imaging
Loma Linda University Medical Center, Loma Linda, CA, USA

BICENTENNIAL
1807
WILEY
2007
BICENTENNIAL

John Wiley & Sons, Ltd

Email (for orders and customer service enquiries): cs-books@wiley.co.uk
Visit our Home Page on www.wiley.com

Reprinted September 2008, December 2009, September 2010

Other Wiley Editorial Offices

John Wiley & Sons Inc., 111 River Street, Hoboken, NJ 07030, USA

Jossey-Bass, 989 Market Street, San Francisco, CA 94103-1741, USA

Wiley-VCH Verlag GmbH, Boschstr. 12, D-69469 Weinheim, Germany

John Wiley & Sons Australia Ltd, 33 Park Road, Milton, Queensland 4064, Australia

John Wiley & Sons (Asia) Pte Ltd, 2 Clementi Loop #02-01, Jin Xing Distripark, Singapore 129809

John Wiley & Sons Canada Ltd, 6045 Freemont Blvd, Mississauga, Ontario, L5R 4J3

Anniversary Logo Design: Richard J. Pacifico

Library of Congress Cataloging-in-Publication Data

Pai, Ramdas G.
  Echocardiography board review : 400 multiple choice questions with discussion / Ramdas G. Pai and Padmini
Varadarajan.
    p. ; cm.
  ISBN 978-0-470-51822-9 (alk. paper)
  1. Echocardiography—Examinations, questions, etc.   I. Varadarajan, Padmini.   II. Title.
  [DNLM: 1. Echocardiography—Examination Questions. WG 18.2 P142e 2007]
  RC683.5.U5P32 2007
  616.1′2075430076—dc22

                                                                          2007040629

British Library Cataloguing in Publication Data

A catalogue record for this book is available from the British Library

ISBN 978-0-470-51822-9 (P/B)

Typeset in 9.5/13 pt Bembo by Integra Software Services Pvt. Ltd, Pondicherry, India.
Printed and bound in Great Britain by CPI Antony Rowe, Chippenham, Wiltshire.

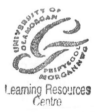

Contents

Preface

The *Echocardiography Board Review* is written for the primary purpose of helping candidates prepare for the National Board of Echocardiography and should be helpful both to the cardiologists and anesthesiologists preparing for this certification process. At the time of its writing, there were no other published works available that comprehensively dealt with the material covered in these examinations in a question, answer and discussion format. The authors have used this format in teaching echocardiography to cardiology fellows in training. One of the main impetuses for initiating this work was the request by many of the trainees and prospective echocardiography examination candidates to write such material. Similar requests have also come from echocardiography technicians preparing for their certification examination. There are 400 well-thought-out questions in this review book. The questions address practically all areas of echocardiography including applied ultrasound physics, practical hydrodynamics, imaging techniques, valvular heart disease, myocardial diseases, congenital heart disease, noninvasive hemodynamics, surgical echocardiography, etc. Each question is followed by several answers to choose from. The discussion addresses not only the rationale behind picking the right choice, but fills in information around the topic under discussion such that important key concepts are clearly driven. This would not only help in the preparation for the examinations, but also give a clear understanding of various echocardiographic techniques, applications and the disease processes they address.

This review would be helpful not only to the prospective examinees in echocardiography, but to all students of echocardiography in training, not only in cardiology and anesthesia training programs in this country but internationally as well. This does not take the place of a standard textbook of echocardiography, but complements the textbook reading by bringing out the salient concepts in a clear fashion. The questions on applied physics, quantitative Doppler and images are of particular value. There are over 200 still images representing most of the key areas and these will improve the diagnostic abilities of the reviewer.

We feel this book will meet the need felt by students of echocardiography in not only preparing for examinations but clearly enhancing the understanding of the subject in an easy-to-read manner. The authors are grateful to many of the trainees who expressed the need for such work and pressured us to write one.

Chapter 1

1. The speed of sound in tissues is:
   A. Roughly 1540 m/s
   B. Roughly 1540 km/s
   C. Roughly 1540 cm/s
   D. Roughly 1540 m/min

2. The mitral flow measurements in a 62–year–old man are: left ventricular (LV) isovolumic relaxation time (IVRT) 50 ms, E/A ratio 1.5 and E–wave deceleration time 140 ms. This is suggestive of:
   A. Normal left atrial (LA) pressure
   B. Abnormal LV relaxation
   C. High LA pressure
   D. None of the above

3. The frame rate increases with:
   A. Increasing the depth
   B. Reducing sector angle
   C. Increasing line density
   D. Adding color Doppler to B–mode imaging

4. The mitral flow measurements in a 1–year–old child are: LV IVRT 50 ms, E/A ratio 2.5 and E–wave deceleration time 120 ms. This is:
   A. Normal
   B. Suggestive of abnormal LV relaxation
   C. Suggestive of high LA pressure
   D. Is pseudonormal

5. Determination of regurgitant orifice area by the proximal isovelocity surface area (PISA) method is based on:
   A. Law of conservation of mass
   B. Law of conservation of energy
   C. Law of conservation of momentum
   D. Jet momentum analysis

6. In which situation can you not use the simplified Bernoulli equation to derive the pressure gradient?
   A. Peak instantaneous gradient across a nonobstructed mitral valve
   B. Peak gradient across a severely stenotic aortic valve

C. Mean gradient across a severely stenotic aortic valve

D. Mean gradient across a stenotic tricuspid valve

7. Which of the following resolutions changes with increasing field depth?
    A. Axial resolution
    B. Lateral resolution

8. With a fixed-focus transducer with crystal diameter 20 mm and wavelength 2.5 mm, what is the depth of the focus?
    A. 40 m
    B. 30 mm
    C. 40 mm
    D. 4 m

9. A sonographer adjusts the ultrasound machine to double the depth of view from 5 cm to 10 cm. If sector angle is reduced to keep the frame rate constant, which of the following has changed?
    A. Axial resolution
    B. Temporal resolution
    C. Lateral resolution
    D. The wavelength

10. Which of the following properties of a reflected wave is most important in the genesis of a two-dimensional image?
    A. Amplitude
    B. Period
    C. Pulse repetition period
    D. Pulse duration

11. Increasing depth will change all of the following except:
    A. Pulse duration
    B. Pulse repetition period
    C. Pulse repetition frequency
    D. Duty factor

12. The two-dimensional images are produced because of this phenomenon when the ultrasound reaches the tissue:
    A. Refraction
    B. Backscatter
    C. Specular reflection
    D. Transmission

13. Attenuation of ultrasound as it travels to the tissue is increased by:
    A. Greater depth
    B. Lower transducer frequency
    C. Blood rather than soft tissue like muscle
    D. Bone more than air

14. The half-intensity depth is a measure of:
    A. Ultrasound attenuation in tissue
    B. Half the wall thickness in mm
    C. Coating on the surface of the transducer
    D. Half the ultrasound beam width

15. What is the highest pulse repetition frequency (PRF) of a 3 MHz pulsed wave transducer imaging at a depth of 7 cm?
    A. 21 000 Hz
    B. 2 333 Hz
    C. 11 000 Hz
    D. 2.1 million Hz

16. Examples of continuous wave imaging include:
    A. Two-dimensional image
    B. Volumetric scanner-acquired LV image
    C. Color flow imaging
    D. Nonimaging Doppler probe (Pedoff)

17. Which of the following manipulations will increase the frame rate?
    A. Increase depth
    B. Increase transmit frequency
    C. Decrease sector angle
    D. Increase transmit power

18. The lateral resolution increases with:
    A. Decreasing transducer diameter
    B. Reducing power
    C. Beam focusing
    D. Reducing transmit frequency

19. Axial resolution can be improved by which of the following manipulations?
    A. Reduce beam diameter
    B. Beam focusing
    C. Reduce gain
    D. Increase transmit frequency

20. Type of sound used in medical imaging is:
    A. Ultrasound
    B. Infrasound
    C. Audible sound

Answers for chapter 1

1. **Answer: A.**
Hence travel time at a depth of 15 cm is roughly 0.1 ms one way (154 000 cm/s or 154 cm/ms or 15 cm per 0.1 ms) or 0.2 ms to and fro. This is independent of transducer frequency and depends only on the medium of transmission.

2. **Answer: C.**
High LA pressure. Normal IVRT in adults is 70–100 ms, E/A ratio is about 1 and E-wave deceleration time is 160–250 ms. High LA pressure shortens IVRT and E-wave deceleration time and increases early LV filling. Abnormal LV relaxation has exactly the opposite effect on the mitral flow profile. Very young children may have a pattern mimicking high LA pressure because of superefficient LV relaxation, which promotes early LV filling.

3. **Answer: B.**
Reducing the sector angle will reduce the time required to complete a frame by reducing the number of scan lines. This increases the temporal resolution. Decreasing depth will increase the frame rate as well. Adding color Doppler will reduce the frame rate.

4. **Answer: A.**
This is normal and results from a very efficient relaxation process, which facilitates early diastolic LV filling. Rapid E-wave deceleration results in physiological S3. And also, as most of the filling occurs in early diastole, children are able to tolerate rapid heart rates and loss of atrial kick without much of a problem. In other words, efficient relaxation mimics high LA pressure in terms of mitral inflow pattern.

5. **Answer: A.**
The law of conservation of mass is the basis of the continuity equation. As the flow rate at the PISA surface and the regurgitant orifice are the same, dividing this by the velocity at the regurgitant orifice obtained by continuous wave Doppler gives the effective regurgitant area (regurgitant flow rate in cm^3/s divided by flow velocity in cm/s equals effective regurgitant area in cm^2).

6. **Answer: A.**
In a nonobstructed mitral valve, significant energy is expended in accelerating the flow (flow acceleration). As viscous losses in this situation are minimal, the other two components (flow acceleration and convective acceleration) of the Bernoulli equation have to be taken into account. In the simplified Bernoulli equation, the flow acceleration component is ignored. Put simply, when you deal with low-velocity signals from pulsatile flows, the simplified Bernoulli equation does not describe the pressure flow relationship accurately.

7. **Answer: B.**
Lateral resolution depends on beam width, which increases at increasing depths. Axial resolution depends on spatial pulse length, which is a function of transducer frequency, pulse duration and propagation velocity in the medium.

8. **Answer: C.**
   Depth of focus equals crystal diameter squared divided by wavelength multiplied by 4. In this situation, $400/10 = 40$ mm.

9. **Answer: C.**
   Lateral resolution diminishes at depths due to beam divergence. Frame rate determines the temporal resolution. Wavelength is a function of the transducer and is independent of depth and frame rate adjustments.

10. **Answer: A.**
    Amplitude or strength of the reflected beam and its temporal registration, which determines depth registration.

11. **Answer: A.**
    Pulse duration is the characteristic of the pulse and does not change with depth. Increasing depth will reduce pulse repetition period, frequency and hence the duty factor.

12. **Answer: B.**
    Backscatter or diffuse reflection produces most of the clinical images. Specular reflection reaches the transducer only when the incident angle is 90° to the surface, which is not the case in most of the images produced. Refracted and transmitted ultrasounds do not come back to the transducer.

13. **Answer: A.**
    Attenuation is the loss of ultrasound energy as it travels through the tissue and is caused by absorption and random scatter. It is greater with longer travel path length as it has to go through more tissue. Attenuation is greater at higher frequencies due to smaller wavelength. Attenuation is greatest for air followed by bone, soft tissue and water.

14. **Answer: A.**
    It is a measure of attenuation and reflects the depth at which the ultrasound energy is reduced by half. It is given by the formula: 6 cm/frequency in MHz. For example, for an ultrasound frequency of 3 MHz the half-intensity depth is 2 cm, and for 6 MHz it is 1 cm.

15. **Answer: C.**
    The PRF is independent of transducer frequency and only determined by time of flight, which is the total time taken by ultrasound in the body in both directions. Ultrasound can travel 154 000 cm in a second at a travel speed of 1540 m/s. In other words, at 1 cm depth (2 cm travel distance) the technical limit to the number of pulses that can be sent is 77 000 per second (Hz). Hence the PRF equals 77 000/depth in cm.

16. **Answer: D.**
    Pedoff is a continuous wave Doppler modality for velocity recording. All other modalities utilize the pulsed wave technique where each of the crystals performs both transmit and receive functions.

17. **Answer: C.**
    Increase in frame rate occurs with reducing sector angle and depth. It is independent of transmit frequency and power.

18. **Answer: C.**

Focusing increases lateral resolution. Increasing transducer diameter and increasing frequency also increase lateral resolution.

19. **Answer: D.**

Increasing the transmit frequency will reduce the wavelength and hence the spatial pulse length. This will increase the PRF and the axial resolution. Beam diameter and focusing have no effect on axial resolution.

20. **Answer: A.**

Typical frequency is 2–30 MHz: 2–7 MHz for cardiac imaging, 10 MHz for intra-cardiac echocardiography and 20–30 MHz for intravascular imaging. Ultrasound in the 100–400 MHz range is used for acoustic microscopy. Frequency $> 20\,000$ Hz is ultrasound.

Chapter 2

21. Doppler shift is typically in:
    A. Ultrasound range
    B. Infrasound range
    C. Audible range

22. Duty factor refers to:
    A. Power the transducer can generate
    B. Range of frequencies the transducer is capable of
    C. Physical properties of the damping material
    D. Fraction of time the transducer is emitting ultrasound

23. Duty factor increases with:
    A. Increasing gain
    B. Increasing pulse duration
    C. Decreasing pulse repetition frequency (PRF)
    D. Decreasing dynamic range

24. Which of the following will increase the PRF?
    A. Reducing depth
    B. Decreasing transducer frequency
    C. Reducing sector angle
    D. Reducing filter

25. Persistence will have this effect on the image:
    A. Smoothing of a two-dimensional image
    B. Better resolution
    C. Eliminating artifacts
    D. Spuriously reducing wall thickness

26. Aliasing occurs in this type of imaging:
    A. Pulsed wave Doppler
    B. Continuous wave Doppler
    C. None of the above
    D. All of the above

27. The Nyquist limit at a PRF of 1000 Hz is:
    A. 500 Hz
    B. 1000 Hz
    C. 2000 Hz
    D. Cannot calculate

28. The Nyquist limit can be increased by:
    A. Increasing the PRF
    B. Reducing the PRF
    C. Neither

29. The Nyquist limit can also be increased by:
    A. Increasing transducer frequency
    B. Reducing transducer frequency
    C. Reducing filter
    D. None of the above

30. Aliasing can be reduced by:
    A. Decreasing the depth
    B. Increasing the PRF
    C. Reducing the transducer frequency
    D. Changing to continuous wave Doppler
    E. All of the above

31. What is the purpose of the depth or time gain compensation process adjusted by the echo cardiographer and performed in an ultrasound's receiver?
    A. Corrects for attenuation and makes the image uniformly bright
    B. Eliminates image artifacts
    C. Eliminates aliasing
    D. None of the above

32. Which of the following increases the Nyquist limit?
    A. Increasing the depth
    B. Reducing the sample volume depth
    C. Increasing the transducer frequency
    D. None of the above

33. The maximum Doppler shift that can be displayed without aliasing with a PRF of 10 kHz is:
    A. 5 kHz
    B. 10 kHz
    C. Depends on depth
    D. Cannot be determined

34. The PRF is influenced by:
    A. Transducer frequency
    B. Depth of imaging
    C. Both
    D. Neither

35. Two identical structures appear on an ultrasound scan. One is real and the other is an artifact, the artifact being deeper than the real structure. What is this artifact called?
    A. Shadowing
    B. Ghosting

C. Speed error artifact

D. Mirror image

36. What is determined by the medium through which sound travels?

    A. Wavelength

    B. Speed

    C. Wavelength and speed

    D. None of the above

37. Image quality on an ultrasound scan is dark throughout? What is the first best step to take?

    A. Increase output power

    B. Increase receiver gain

    C. Change to a higher frequency transducer

    D. Decrease receiver gain

38. All of the following will improve temporal resolution except:

    A. Decreasing line density

    B. Decreasing sector angle

    C. Increasing frame rate

    D. Multifocusing

39. Sound travels faster in a medium with which of the following characteristics?

    A. High density, low stiffness

    B. Low density, high stiffness

    C. High density, high stiffness

    D. Low density, low stiffness

40. Which of the following is associated with continuous wave Doppler compared to pulsed wave Doppler?

    A. Aliasing

    B. Range specificity

    C. Ability to record higher velocities

    D. All of the above

Answers for chapter 2

21. **Answer: C.**
Doppler shift resulting from moving blood is generally audible. Audible frequency is 20–20 000 Hz.

22. **Answer: D.**
It is pulse duration divided by pulse repetition period. Typical value for two-dimensional imaging is 0.1–1% and for Doppler it is 0.5–5%. Example for a 2 MHz transducer: the wavelength in tissue is 0.75 mm (period = 0.5 μs); if two periods are in a pulse then pulse duration is 1 μs and if PRF is 1000 Hz (pulse repetition period will be 1 ms or 1000 μs) then the duty factor is 0.1%.

23. **Answer: B.**
Proportional to pulse duration if the PRP is constant. If pulse duration is constant, decreasing the PRF will reduce the duty factor. Gain and dynamic range have no effect on duty factor.

24. **Answer: A.**
Reducing depth reduces time of flight of ultrasound in the body and hence will increase the PRF.

25. **Answer: A.**
Persistence is the process of keeping the prior frames on the display console and will smoothen the image. This reduces random noise and strengthens the signal. However, fast-moving structures can produce artifacts and make the structures look thicker than they are. Some of the other smoothing algorithms include interdigitation and blooming to reduce the spoking appearance produced by the scan lines.

26. **Answer: A.**
Aliasing or wrap-around occurs when the Nyquist limit or upper limit of measurable velocity is reached. The Nyquist limit is determined by the PRF. Spectral pulsed wave Doppler and color flow imaging are pulsed wave modalities.

27. **Answer: A.**
Nyquist limit = PRF/2.

28. **Answer: A.**
Nyquist limit = PRF/2.

29. **Answer: B.**
Reducing transducer frequency will increase aliasing velocity and reduces range ambiguity. For a given detected Doppler shift, the lower the transducer frequency, the higher is the measured velocity. V in cm/s = $(77F_d$ in kHz$)/F_o$ in MHz for an incident angle of zero, where F_d is the Doppler shift and F_o is the transmitting frequency.

30. **Answer: E.**
All of the above.

31. **Answer: A.**

    It is postprocessing, which adjusts for loss of ultrasound that occurs at increasing depths.

32. **Answer: B.**

    The Nyquist limit is determined by the PRF and PRF = 77 000/depth in cm. Hence decreasing the sample volume depth will increase the PRF, which in turn will increase the Nyquist limit.

33. **Answer: A.**

    The Nyquist limit is PRF/2. Hence, a Doppler shift of >5 kHz in this case will cause aliasing. Depth influences the PRF.

34. **Answer: B.**

    The PRF is influenced by pulse duration and time need for ultrasound to travel in tissue. Increasing depth will increase the time spent in the body.

35. **Answer: D.**

    Mirror image artifact is a type of artifact where the artifact is always deeper than the real structure and occurs because of the structure or the surface between the two functioning as a mirror.

36. **Answer: C.**

    Speed is determined only by the medium through which sound is traveling. For a given frequency, speed will determine the wavelength: the greater the speed, the longer the wavelength. Period is the time taken for one cycle and is determined by frequency and is independent of the transmission medium.

37. **Answer: A.**

    The first best action to take is to increase output power. This will brighten the overall image. If the image is still dark, then the receiver gain should be increased.

38. **Answer: D.**

    Multifocusing will decrease temporal resolution by decreasing the frame rate, whereas all the others will improve temporal resolution by facilitating an increase in the frame rate.

39. **Answer: B.**

    Sound travels faster in a medium with low density and high stiffness.

40. **Answer: C.**

    Aliasing and range specificity are properties of pulsed wave Doppler. Continuous wave Doppler is associated with range ambiguity. Continuous wave Doppler will also permit recording of higher velocities than pulsed wave Doppler, as it is not limited by the PRF.

Chapter 3

41. As frequency increases, backscatter strength:
    A. Decreases
    B. Increases
    C. Does not change
    D. Refracts

42. If an echo arrives 39 μs after a pulse has been emitted, at what depth should the reflecting object be on the scan line?
    A. 3 cm
    B. 6 cm
    C. 1 cm
    D. None of the above

43. The Doppler shift produced by an object moving at a speed of 1 m/s towards the transducer emitting ultrasound at 2 MHz would be:
    A. 2.6 kHz
    B. 1.3 kHz
    C. 1 MHz
    D. 200 Hz

44. In the above example, the reflected ultrasound will have a frequency of:
    A. 2 002 600 Hz
    B. 1 998 700 Hz
    C. 1 000 000 Hz
    D. 2 MHz

45. Reflected ultrasound from an object moving away from the sound source will have a frequency:
    A. Higher than original sound
    B. Lower than the original sound
    C. Same as the original sound
    D. Variable, depending on source of sound and velocity of the moving object

46. Reflected ultrasound from an object moving perpendicular to the sound source will have a frequency:
    A. Higher than original sound
    B. Lower than the original sound
    C. Same as the original sound
    D. Variable, depending on source of sound and velocity of the moving object

47. Doppler shift frequency is independent of:
    A. Operating frequency
    B. Doppler angle
    C. Propagation speed
    D. Amplitude

48. On a continuous wave Doppler display, amplitude is represented by:
    A. Brightness of the signal
    B. Vertical extent of the signal
    C. Width of the signal
    D. None of the above

49. Doppler signals from the myocardium, compared to those from the blood pool, display:
    A. Lower velocity
    B. Greater amplitude
    C. Both of the above
    D. None of the above

50. Doing which of the following modifications to the Doppler processing will allow myocardial velocities to be recorded selectively compared to blood pool velocities?
    A. A band pass filter that allows low velocities
    B. A band pass filter that allows high amplitude signals
    C. Both
    D. Neither

51. If the propagation speed is 1.6 mm/µs and the pulse round trip time is 5 µs, the distance to the reflector is:
    A. 8 mm
    B. 4 mm
    C. 10 mm
    D. Cannot be determined

52. How long after a pulse is sent out by a transducer does an echo from an object at a depth of 5 cm return?
    A. 13 µs
    B. 65 µs
    C. 5 µs
    D. Cannot be determined

53. For soft tissues, the attenuation coefficient at 3 MHz is:
    A. 1 dB/cm
    B. 6 dB/cm
    C. 1.5 dB/cm
    D. 3 dB/cm

54. If the density of a medium is 1000 kg/m³ and the propagation speed is 1540 m/s, the impedance is:
    A. 1 540 000 rayls
    B. 770 000 rayls

C. 3 080 000 rayls

D. Cannot be determined

55. If the propagation speed through medium 2 is greater than the propagation speed through medium 1 the transmission angle will be ——— the incidence angle.
    A. Smaller
    B. Larger
    C. Equal to
    D. Cannot be determined

56. If amplitude is doubled, intensity is:
    A. Halved
    B. Quadrupled
    C. Remains the same
    D. Tripled

57. If both power and area are doubled, intensity is:
    A. Doubled
    B. Unchanged
    C. Halved
    D. Tripled

58. Flow resistance in a vessel depends on:
    A. Vessel length
    B. Vessel radius
    C. Blood viscosity
    D. All of the above
    E. None of the above

59. Flow resistance decreases with an increase in:
    A. Vessel length
    B. Vessel radius
    C. Blood viscosity
    D. None of the above

60. Flow resistance depends most strongly on:
    A. Vessel length
    B. Vessel radius
    C. Blood viscosity
    D. All of the above

Answers for chapter 3

41. **Answer: B.**
    Smaller wavelengths are more readily reflected compared to longer wavelengths.

42. **Answer: A.**
    Ultrasound takes 6.5 ms to travel 1 cm in the tissues assuming a speed of 1540 m/s. 39 ms is travel time for 6 cm; hence the object is 3 cm deep.

43. **Answer: A.**
    $F_d = (2F_o V\cos$ of incident angle$)/C$ where F_d is the Doppler shift, V is the velocity and C is the speed of sound in the medium. In this example, $F_d = (2 \times 2\,000\,000 \times 1 \times 1)/1540 = 2600$ Hz or 2.6 kHz. For each MHz of emitted sound, a target velocity of 1 m/s will produce a Doppler shift of 1.3 kHz.

44. **Answer: A.**
    As the object is moving directly towards the source of sound, the reflected sound will have a higher frequency and will equal F_o plus F_d.

45. **Answer: B.**
    Object moving away will produce a negative Doppler shift.

46. **Answer: C.**
    As the cosine of the incident angle of 90° is zero, the Doppler shift is zero (please look at Doppler equation in question 43). Because of the this angle dependence of the Doppler shift, the angle between the direction of motion of the object and the ultrasound beam has to be as close to zero as possible to record the true Doppler shift and hence the true velocity. Cosine of 0° is 1, cosine of 20° is 0.94 and cosine of 90° is 0. Angle correction is generally not used for intracardiac flows because of the three-dimensional nature of intracardiac flows and fallacies of assumed angles in contrast to flow in tubular structures.

47. **Answer: D.**
    Please look up the Doppler equation in question 43.

48. **Answer: A.**
    Amplitude is strength of the returning signal. Vertical extent is the velocity of the object and horizontal axis is the time axis and gives distribution or timing of the signal in the cardiac cycle.

49. **Answer: C.**
    Myocardium produces stronger or higher amplitude signals that have lower velocities compared to the blood pool.

50. **Answer: C.**
    In contrast, blood pool signals are higher velocity and lower amplitude.

51. **Answer: B.**
    The distance to the reflector is calculated by the range equation. The formula is ½ (propagation speed (mm/µs) × round trip time (µs)). So, solving the equation gives ½ (1.6 × 5) = 4 mm.

52. **Answer: B.**

    The round trip travel time for 1 cm is 13 μs. Hence for an object at 5 cm the travel time is 13 μs × 5 = 65 μs.

53. **Answer: C.**

    Attenuation coefficient in soft tissue is equivalent to ½ × frequency (MHz). In the above question ½ × 3 = 1.5 dB/cm. Multiplying this by the path length (cm) yields the attenuation (dB).

54. **Answer: A.**

    Impedance describes the relationship between acoustic pressure and the speed of particle vibrations in a sound wave. It is equal to the density of a medium × propagation speed. Solving the equation gives 1000 × 1540 = 1 540 000 rayls. Impedance is increased if the density of the medium is increased or the propagation speed is increased.

55. **Answer: B.**

    When the propagation speed in medium 2 is greater than medium 1 the transmission angle will be greater than the incidence angle.

56. **Answer: B.**

    Intensity is the rate at which energy passes through a unit area. Intensity is equal to amplitude squared. Hence, if amplitude is doubled, intensity is quadrupled.

57. **Answer: B.**

    Intensity is given by the equation Power (mW)/Area (cm^2). Hence if both power and area are doubled, intensity will remain the same.

58. **Answer: D.**

    Flow resistance is $= 8 \times$ length $\times$ viscosity/$\pi \times$ radius^4.

59. **Answer: B.**

    Flow resistance decreases with an increase in the vessel radius. Please refer to question 58 for the relationship. Resistance to flow and hence flow rate for a given driving pressure depends upon radius, length and viscosity.

60. **Answer: B.**

    Flow resistance is inversely related to radius^4, hence it is most strongly related to the vessel radius.

Chapter 4

61. Volumetric flow rate decreases with an increase in:
    A. Pressure difference
    B. Vessel radius
    C. Vessel length
    D. Blood viscosity
    E. Vessel length and blood viscosity

62. Which of the following on a color Doppler display is represented in real time?
    A. Gray-scale anatomy
    B. Flow direction
    C. Doppler spectrum
    D. Gray-scale anatomy and flow direction
    E. All of the above

63. Approximately how many pulses are required to obtain one line of color Doppler information?
    A. 1
    B. 100
    C. 10
    D. 10 000

64. Multiple focus is not used in color Doppler imaging because:
    A. It would not improve the image
    B. Doppler transducers cannot focus
    C. Frame rates would be too low
    D. None of the above

65. Widening the color box on the display will ———— the frame rate.
    A. Increase
    B. No change
    C. Decrease
    D. Cannot be determined

66. The simplified Bernoulli equation is inapplicable under the following circumstances:
    A. Serial stenotic lesions
    B. Long, tubular lesions
    C. Both
    D. None of the above

67. The Bernoulli equation is an example of:
    A. Law of conservation of mass
    B. Law of conservation of energy
    C. Law of conservation of momentum
    D. None of the above

68. The continuity equation is an example of:
    A. Law of conservation of mass
    B. Law of conservation of energy
    C. Law of conservation of momentum
    D. None of the above

69. Effective regurgitant orifice area by the proximal isovelocity surface area (PISA) method is an example of:
    A. Law of conservation of mass
    B. Law of conservation of energy
    C. Law of conservation of momentum
    D. None of the above

70. Doppler calculation of aortic valve area is an example of:
    A. Law of conservation of mass
    B. Law of conservation of energy
    C. Law of conservation of momentum
    D. None of the above

71. Calculation of right ventricular systolic pressure from the tricuspid regurgitation velocity signal is an example of:
    A. Law of conservation of mass
    B. Law of conservation of energy
    C. Law of conservation of momentum
    D. None of the above

72. Color flow jet area of mitral regurgitation depends upon:
    A. Amount of regurgitation alone
    B. Driving pressure and the regurgitant volume
    C. Presence of aortic regurgitation
    D. Degree of mitral stenosis

73. Factors influencing mitral regurgitation jet volume also include:
    A. Proximity of left atrial wall
    B. Heart rate
    C. Gain setting
    D. Filter setting
    E. Left atrial size
    F. All of the above

74. Amount of mitral regurgitation depends upon:
    A. Regurgitant orifice size
    B. Driving pressure

C. Duration of systole

D. All of the above

75. Hemodynamic impact of a given volumetric severity of mitral regurgitation (MR) is increased by:

A. Nondilated left atrium

B. Left ventricular hypertrophy

C. Presence of concomitant aortic regurgitation

D. All of the above

E. None of the above

76. Which feature is consistent with severe MR:

A. Jet size to left atrial area ratio of 0.5

B. The PISA radius of 1.2 cm at an aliasing velocity of 50 cm/s

C. Effective regurgitant orifice area of 0.7 cm^2

D. All of the above

E. None of the above

77. When using a fixed-focus probe this parameter cannot be changed by the sonographer:

A. Pulse repetition period

B. Pulse repetition frequency

C. Amplitude

D. Wavelength

78. The following signal was obtained from the apical view in a 45-year-old man with a systolic murmur. What is the most likely origin of this signal?

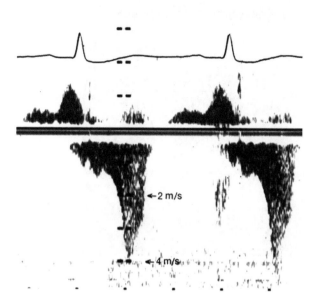

A. Mitral valve prolapse with late systolic MR

B. Rheumatic MR

    C. Hyperdynamic left ventricle with cavity obliteration

    D. Subaortic membrane

79. Continuous wave signal from the apical view. The image is suggestive of:

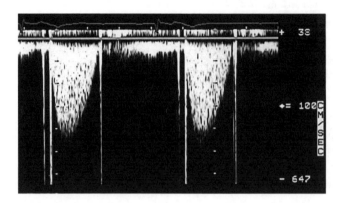

    A. Moderate aortic stenosis

    B. Severe aortic stenosis

    C. Mitral regurgitation

    D. Prosthetic aortic valve obstruction

80. The signal obtained from the right parasternal view is suggestive of:

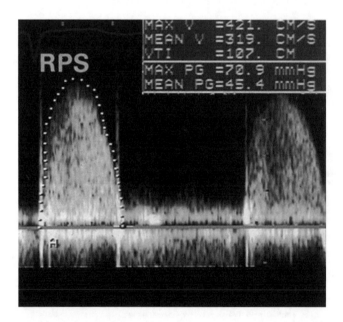

    A. Severe MR

    B. Severe aortic stenosis

    C. Severe aortic regurgitation

    D. Severe pulmonary stenosis

Answers for chapter 4

61. **Answer: E.**

    Volume flow rate = pressure difference $\times \pi \times$ diameter^4/128 $\times$ length $\times$ viscosity. Hence with an increase in length and viscosity the volume flow rate will decrease. An increase in driving pressure and radius will increase the flow rate.

62. **Answer: D.**

63. **Answer: C.**

64. **Answer: C.**

    Combination of multiple pulses needed for a scan line, multiple focusing and need for some width for color flow display box will markedly reduce frame rate.

65. **Answer: C.**

    By increasing the number of scan lines per box.

66. **Answer: C.**

    For the simplified Bernoulli equation to work, the lesion has to be a discrete stenosis. In serial lesions, there may be incomplete recovery of pressure and flow area may be smaller than the anatomic area before the second lesion is encountered. Hence the pressure gradient at the first orifice estimated by the simplified Bernoulli equation will be higher than the actual gradient because of the unmeasured kinetic energy between two orifices. Hence, the total gradient is not the sum of $4V^2$ at the two orifices. For long tubular lesions, viscous forces predominate and Poiseulle's equation would be applicable to analyze the pressure–flow relationship.

67. **Answer: B.**

    Describes the relationship between different types of energies as potential (pressure), kinetic (flow) and viscous forces along a flow stream. Energy can be transformed from one form to the other, but cannot be destroyed or created.

68. **Answer: A.**

    Says that mass cannot be destroyed and hence flow rates at different locations in a flow stream are the same at a given point in time.

69. **Answer: A.**

70. **Answer: A.**

71. **Answer: B.**

72. **Answer: B.**

    Driving pressure influences the jet area independent of regurgitant volume as jet area is proportional to the kinetic energy imparted to the jet, which is proportional to the jet, volume and also the driving pressure. Increase in driving pressure will also increase the regurgitant volume for a given regurgitant orifice.

73. **Answer: F.**

    All of these affect the jet size. Compared to the central jet, a wall-hugging jet is about 50% smaller for a given volume and a nonwall-hugging eccentric jet may be larger due to the

Coanda effect where the jet spreads due to pull towards the wall. Lower gains and higher filter settings reduce jet size. At a faster heart rate, due to reduced jet sampling the jet size may be underestimated. Free jet (receiving chamber at least five times the jet size) has a larger size compared to a contained jet entering a smaller chamber.

74. **Answer: D.**

Regurgitant volume is directly proportional to the regurgitant orifice size, driving pressure and the time over which regurgitation occurs.

75. **Answer: D.**

Noncompliant left atrium as well as left ventricular hypertrophy will increase the hemo-dynamic impact of MR. Presence of aortic regurgitation will add another source of volume load on the left ventricle. Other factors that may have an adverse impact include anemia, fever and acuteness of onset.

76. **Answer: D.**

All of the above. Correlates of severe MR include MR jet area of ≥ 8 cm^2, jet to left atrial area of ≥ 0.4, vena contracta diameter of ≥ 7 mm, effective regurgitant orifice area of ≥ 0.4 cm^2 or ≥ 40 mm^2 and systolic flow reversal in the pulmonary veins. It has to be kept in mind that wall-hugging jets are smaller for a given regurgitant volume and the effective orifice area may not be constant during systole.

77. **Answer: D.**

The wavelength cannot be changed by the sonographer when using a fixed-focus probe.

78. **Answer: C.**

Left ventricular cavity obliteration. The thin dagger suggests a diminishing flow area in late systole. Though this can occur on left ventriclular outflow obstruction due to SAM, the peak tends to be a little earlier at this gradient. A very late peaking signal is suggestive of cavity obliteration. This is a complete velocity profile and flow acceleration is clearly seen. In mitral valve prolapse, an incomplete signal may give a spurious late peaking signal. Signal profile depends solely on the left ventricular to left atrial pressure gradient in MR; only the signal intensity depends on the instantaneous regurgitant flow rate, which determines the number of scatterers.

79. **Answer: D.**

Note the aortic valve opening and closing clicks. There are two opening clicks indicating dyssynchronous opening of a bileaflet mechanical aortic valve and a mid-peaking systolic velocity 4.5 m/s corresponding to a peak gradient of 80 mmHg. The gradient in the prosthetic valve depends upon valve size, valve type and flow.

80. **Answer: B.**

Severe aortic stenosis. This is a signal occupying the ejection phase and directed to the right shoulder, which is typical of aortic stenosis. A flail posterior mitral leaflet may cause a jet directed in this direction but is holosystolic starting with the QRS complex. The signal of aortic regurgitation is diastolic. The pulmonary stenosis signal is recorded best from the left parasternal, apical or subcostal locations.

Chapter 5

Questions

81. The Doppler signal is consistent with:

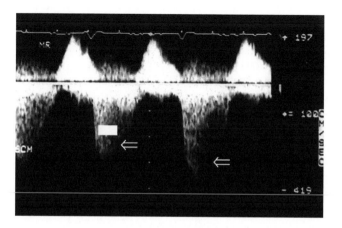

   A. Severe aortic regurgitation and moderate aortic stenosis
   B. Severe mitral stenosis
   C. Acute severe mitral regurgitation
   D. Ventricular septal defect

82. Pulse duration is affected by:
   A. Source of ultrasound
   B. Transmission medium
   C. Both
   D. Neither

83. The pulse repetition frequency (PRF) is affected by:
   A. Source of ultrasound
   B. Transmission medium
   C. Both
   D. Neither

84. What happens to the PRF when imaging depth is increased?
   A. Increases
   B. Decreases
   C. Does not change
   D. Effect is variable

85. By increasing the PRF, the axial resolution:
    A. Increases
    B. Decreases
    C. Does not change

86. Imaging at depth affects:
    A. Axial resolution
    B. Lateral resolution
    C. Neither
    D. Both

87. Reducing the transducer footprint will affect:
    A. Lateral resolution
    B. Temporal resolution
    C. Axial resolution
    D. None of the above

88. Increasing the transmit power will:
    A. Decrease sensitivity
    B. Increase lateral resolution
    C. Increase penetration
    D. None of the above

89. Acoustic impedance equals (rayls):
    A. Density in kg/m^3 × speed of sound in m/s
    B. Density in kg/m^3 × transducer frequency in MHz
    C. Depth in meters × transducer frequency in MHz
    D. None of the above

90. Reflection of sound at an interface is affected by:
    A. Specific acoustic impedance
    B. Transducer frequency
    C. Depth
    D. None of the above

91. The most common cause of coronary sinus dilatation is:
    A. Heart failure
    B. Persistent left superior vena cava
    C. Atrial septal defect
    D. None of the above

92. The following data were obtained from a 72-year-old man with a calcified aortic valve: left ventricular outflow tract (LVOT) velocity (V_1) 0.8 m/s, transaortic velocity (V_2) 4 m/s, LVOT diameter 2 cm. The calculated aortic valve area (AVA) is:
    A. $0.4\,cm^2$
    B. $0.6\,cm^2$
    C. $0.8\,cm^2$
    D. $1\,cm^2$

93. The continuity equation is an example of:
    A. Law of conservation of mass
    B. Law of conservation of energy
    C. Law of conservation of momentum
    D. None of the above

94. The most practical value for the development of perfluorocarbon bubbles was to improve:
    A. Contrast on the right side
    B. Stable passage through the transpulmonary bed to improve contrast on the left side
    C. Improve contrast visualization in the hepatic bed
    D. None of the above

95. In a patient with mixed aortic valve disease, the AVA by the Gorlin equation using Fick cardiac output is likely to be:
    A. Less than by the continuity equation
    B. More than by the continuity equation
    C. The same by both methods

96. In a patient with mixed aortic valve disease, the AVA by the Gorlin equation using angiographic cardiac output is likely to be:
    A. Less than by the continuity equation
    B. More than by the continuity equation
    C. The same by both methods

97. The following measurements were obtained from a mitral regurgitant jet:
    Radius of proximal isovelocity surface area $= 1$ cm, aliasing velocity $= 40$ cm/s. The peak regurgitant flow rate equals:
    A. 251 cc/s
    B. 251 cc/min
    C. 125 cc/min
    D. 125 cc/s

98. In the patient above the systemic blood pressure is 120/80 mmHg in the absence of aortic stenosis and the left atrial pressure is 20 mmHg. The effective mitral regurgitant orifice area would be:
    A. 0.7 cm^2
    B. 0.5 cm^2
    C. 1 cm^2
    D. Cannot be calculated

99. This effective regurgitant orifice (ERO) area of 0.5 cm^2 represents:
    A. Mild mitral regurgitation (MR)
    B. Moderate MR
    C. Severe MR
    D. Severity cannot be detected

100. If the patient in question 99 had a blood pressure of 220/90 mmHg with similar proximal isovelocity surface area (PISA) measurements, the ERO area would:
    A. Remain unchanged
    B. Be more
    C. Be less

Answers for chapter 5

81. **Answer: C.**
Acute severe mitral regurgitation (MR). The image shows the classical "V wave cut-off" sign. The rapid deceleration of the MR velocity profile following the peak velocity is due to a rapidly diminishing left ventricular to left atrial (LV–LA) pressure gradient secondary to a large V wave in the left atrium that is a feature of severe MR, especially when it occurs acutely.

82. **Answer: A.**
Source of ultrasound. Speed of ultrasound transmission affects only lengths, not durations.

83. **Answer: A.**
Source of ultrasound. Speed of ultrasound transmission affects only lengths, not the durations or frequency.

84. **Answer: B.**
It decreases because of an increase in time of flight. PRF = 77 000/depth in cm.

85. **Answer: C.**
The PRF does not affect axial resolution. Axial resolution is determined by spatial pulse length, which is mainly determined by wavelength (i.e. ultrasound frequency) and number of cycles in the pulse as transmission speed in biological systems is fairly fixed.

86. **Answer: B.**
Lateral resolution drops because of beam divergence and widening.

87. **Answer: A.**
It will affect beam width and hence the lateral resolution.

88. **Answer: C.**
Penetration increases due to more power. The sensitivity increases, but lateral resolution decreases due to increasing beam width.

89. **Answer: A.**
Average soft tissue impedance is 1 630 000 rayls.

90. **Answer: A.**

91. **Answer: A.**
Heart failure is the common cause of dilatation of the coronary sinus. Although persistent left superior vena cava (SVC) causes dilatation of the coronary sinus, it occurs infrequently. In the absence of heart failure persistent left SVC is the most common cause of enlarged coronary sinus. Dilatation can occur either due to increased flow in the coronary sinus or due to increased right atrial pressure. The other causes include coronary aortic valve fistula and unroofing of the coronary sinus, which causes a left to right shunt, a variant of atrial septal defect.

92. **Answer: B.**

The valve area can be calculated with the continuity equation.

$A_1 V_1$ (LVOT area × LVOT velocity) = $A_2 V_2$ (aortic valve area × aortic velocity).

$A_2 = A_1 V_1 / V_2$. $A_1 = \pi r^2$ (r = LVOT diameter/2) = 3.14 ×1×1 = 3.14 cm^2.

$A_2 = 3.14 \times 0.8/4 = 0.6$ cm^2.

93. **Answer: A.**

States that mass cannot be destroyed and hence flow rates at different locations in a flow stream are the same at a given point in time.

94. **Answer: B.**

The development of perflorocarbon bubbles increased stable passage through the pulmonary bed, so that contrast visualization was better on the left side.

95. **Answer: A.**

The cardiac output by the Fick method is less than the transaortic flow, which is Fick cardiac output + regurgitant volume. Hence the calculation of AVA by Gorlin will underestimate AVA compared to AVA by the continuity equation.

96. **Answer: C.**

Angiographic and Doppler cardiac output would be equal.

97. **Answer: A.**

The regurgitant flow rate is calculated by the formula $2\pi r^2$ × aliasing velocity. This formula assumes a hemispherical geometry. Hence it is vital to optimize the aliasing velocity to maximize the hemisphere of the PISA in all dimensions. Using the formula, peak flow rate = $2\pi r^2$ = 2 × 3.14 ×1×1× 40 = 251.2 cc/s.

98. **Answer: B.**

The LA–LV pressure gradient is 100 mmHg, which corresponds to a peak mitral regurgitant velocity of 5 m/s or 500 cm/s. The ERO area is given by the formula $2\pi r^2$ × aliasing velocity (peak flow rate)/MR velocity. In this patient, peak flow rate = 251 cc/s and ERO is 251/500 = 0.5 cm^2.

99. **Answer: C.**

This patient has severe MR. The ERO is a fairly stable measure of quantitating MR as it represents the defect in the mitral valve coaptation mechanism and is independent of loading conditions. ERO < 0.2 is mild, 0.2–0.4 is moderate and ≥0.4 cm^2 is severe MR.

100. **Answer: C.**

Since the blood pressure is now elevated, the LV–LA pressure gradient is 200 mmHg, giving rise to an MR jet of 7 m/s. The ERO now is 251/700 = 0.3 cm^2. If the ERO were unchanged, the peak flow rate would be increased because of higher driving pressure and the PISA radius would be increased.

Chapter 6

101. An intraoperative trans-esophageal echocardiogram (TEE) revealed mitral regurgitation with the following measurements: regurgitant jet area 4 cm^2, PISA radius 0.8 cm at a Nyquist limit of 50 cm/s at a heart rate of 82 beats/min and arterial blood pressure 80/40 mmHg. This represents:
    A. Mild mitral regurgitation (MR)
    B. Moderate MR
    C. Severe MR

102. For the patient in the above question, if the systolic blood pressure is increased to 145 mmHg, assuming that the effective orifice area is unchanged, then the:
    A. MR jet size will double
    B. MR jet size will not change
    C. MR jet size will more than double

103. For a given regurgitant volume all of the following result in a reduction in the jet size except:
    A. Fast heart rate
    B. Doubling the sector angle
    C. Increasing the imaging depth
    D. Increasing the blood pressure

104. In a patient with severe MR all of the following factors increase its hemodynamic impact except:
    A. Mitral stenosis
    B. Left ventricular hypertrophy
    C. Compliant left atrium
    D. Concomitant aortic regurgitation

105. In a patient undergoing aortic valve replacement (AVR) for aortic stenosis, there was evidence of moderate MR on a preoperative transthoracic echocardiogram. After the AVR, the next step to be taken is:
    A. Replace the mitral valve
    B. Leave the mitral valve alone
    C. Assess for MR with intraoperative TEE, and decide if repair or replacement is needed
    D. None of the above

106. A patient with old inferior wall myocardial infarction (MI) has severe MR with a posterolaterally directed jet in the left atrium. The most likely cause of MR in this patient is:

    A. Flail posterior leaflet

    B. Dilated mitral annulus

    C. Tented or apically tethered posterior mitral leaflet

    D. Tented or apically tethered anterior mitral leaflet

107. Presence of severe aortic regurgitation (AR) in a patient with mitral stenosis is likely to do the following to the calculated mitral valve area by the pressure half-time method:

    A. Overestimate the valve area

    B. Underestimate the valve area

    C. No effect

108. Presence of atrial septal defect (ASD) in a patient with mitral stenosis is likely to do the following to the calculated mitral valve area by the pressure half-time method:

    A. Overestimate the valve area

    B. Underestimate the valve area

    C. No change

109. In a patient with mitral stenosis, the following diastolic flow measurements were obtained: maximal radius of proximal isovelocity surface area (PISA) 0.8 cm at an aliasing velocity of 50 cm/s, inlet angle 120°, peak inflow velocity 2 m/s. The mitral valve area is:

    A. 0.7 cm^2

    B. 1 cm^2

    C. 1.2 cm^2

    D. 1.5 cm^2

110. A patient with mitral stenosis without any MR or AR has a stroke volume of 70 cc/beat, a transmitral flow integral of 50 cm and the mitral valve area is:

    A. 0.7

    B. 1

    C. 1.4

    D. None of the above

111. A patient with MR has a transaortic flow of 70 cc/beat by the left ventricular outflow tract (LVOT) method and a transmitral flow of 112 cc/beat by the mitral annular method. The time velocity integral (TVI) of the MR signal by continuous wave Doppler is 60 cm. The effective regurgitant orifice (ERO) area of this patient is:

    A. 1.5 cm^2

    B. 0.7 cm^2

    C. 0.4 cm^2

    D. 0.2 cm^2

112. For a patient with MR and AR the following measurements were obtained using echo Doppler: flow across the pulmonary valve 75 cc/beat, flow across the mitral valve 120 cc/beat, flow across the aortic valve 90 cc/beat, TVI of MR signal 90 cm, TVI of AR signal 75 cm. The following statement is accurate in this patient:

    A. MR ERO is 0.5 cm^2 and AR ERO is 0.2 cm^2

B. MR ERO is 1.3 cm^2 and AR ERO is 1.2 cm^2

C. Cannot be calculated

113. In a patient with isolated AR the following measurements were obtained: transmitral flow 80 cc/beat, flow across aortic valve 140 cc/beat, TVI of AR signal 100 cm. The AR in this patient is:

A. Mild

B. Moderate

C. Severe

D. Cannot be determined

114. A patient with dilated cardiomyopathy has an end diastolic pulmonary regurgitation (PR) velocity of 2 m/s and the estimated right atrial pressure is 10 mmHg. The following statement is true about this patient:

A. Pulmonary artery (PA) pressure is normal

B. Has mild or moderate pulmonary hypertension

C. Has severe pulmonary hypertension

D. Cannot estimate pulmonary pressure

115. If the patient in question 114 had valvular pulmonary stenosis (PS) with a peak gradient of 36 mmHg, the estimated PA end diastolic pressure would be:

A. 16 mmHg

B. 26 mmHg

C. 36 mmHg

D. 62 mmHg

116. If the patient in question 114 has tricuspid stenosis with a mean diastolic gradient of 8 mmHg across the tricuspid valve, the PA diastolic pressure would be:

A. 26 mmHg

B. 34 mmHg

C. 18 mmHg

D. Cannot be estimated

117. In a patient with valvular PS with right PA branch stenosis, the following measurements were obtained: tricuspid regurgitation (TR) velocity 4 m/s, right atrial (RA) pressure 6 mmHg, systolic velocity across the pulmonary valve 2.5 m/s, velocity across the discrete branch stenosis 2.5 m/s. The systolic pressure in the right pulmonary branch distal to the stenosis is likely to be:

A. 20 mmHg

B. 5 mmHg

C. 70 mmHg

D. Cannot be estimated

118. A 20-year-old patient with a large ventricular septal defect (VSD) underwent PA banding in childhood and was lost to follow-up. A recent echocardiogram revealed the following: peak systolic velocity across the VSD 3 m/s, TR velocity 5 m/s, estimated RA pressure 10 mmHg, cuff blood pressure in the right arm 146/70 mmHg, peak flow velocity across the pulmonary band 4.7 m/s. The following statement is true:

    A. This patient has normal PA pressure

    B. The patient has severe pulmonary hypertension

    C. The patient has features of left ventricular (LV) failure

    D. PA pressure cannot be determined

119. The patient has an LVOT velocity of 1 m/s, TVI of 25 cm, LVOT diameter 2 cm, aortic transvalvular velocity of 1.5 m/s, heart rate 70 beats/min and the cardiac output in this patient is:

    A. 5.5 L

    B. 4.5 L

    C. 6.3 L

    D. Cannot be determined based on the given data

120. A patient with aortic stenosis has an LVOT diameter of 2 cm, LVOT velocity (V_1) 2.5 m/s, transaortic valve velocity (V_2) 5 m/s and two-dimensional examination showed moderate systolic anterior motion of the mitral leaflet. Valvular aortic stenosis in this patient is:

    A. Mild

    B. Moderate

    C. Severe

    D. Cannot be calculated based on given data

Answers for chapter 6

101. **Answer: C.**

Jet area underestimates the severity of MR as the driving pressure is low. The regurgitant flow rate is approximately 200 cc/s. Because of low LV systolic pressure of 80 mmHg, the MR velocity would be in the range of 4 m/s (400 cm/s) assuming an LA pressure of 16 mmHg. Hence, the ERO area would be about 200/400 or 0.5 cm^2. Hence, in an intraoperative setting, it is important to bring up the blood pressure before performing MR quantitation.

102. **Answer: C.**

As the driving pressure across the mitral valve is doubled, the regurgitant volume is doubled, as it is directly proportional to the driving pressure. However jet size is not only dependent on regurgitant volume but also on the kinetic energy imparted to the jet, which depends on jet velocity and, indirectly, the driving pressure. In this patient the jet area would be about three times larger, i.e. 12 cm^2.

103. **Answer: D.**

Underestimation of MR can occur due to undersampling in the setting of low frame rate (increasing sector angle and depth) and high heart rates. Increasing blood pressure will increase the driving pressure across the mitral valve and hence the jet size will increase.

104. **Answer: C.**

A noncompliant left atrium causes a greater rise in left atrial pressure for a given regurgitant volume as it occurs in acute MR. Noncompliant left ventricle and concomitant volume overloads such as aortic regurgitation and anemia increase LV diastolic pressure. In patients with mitral stenosis, the presence of MR increases the transvalvular flow and the gradient.

105. **Answer: C.**

This patient had evidence of moderate MR on the preoperative echocardiogram. In most patients just replacing the aortic valve causes MR to regress. The MR, if functional, regresses with AVR, but MR due to structural pathology is unlikely to regress. The functional MR is due to high driving pressure and increased LV end systolic size. With the relief of the high driving pressure, it is likely to regress. But after the AVR the mitral valve should be assessed intraoperatively to decide on repair versus replacement. There is no clear consensus on decision-making in patients like these.

106. **Answer: C.**

In a patient with inferior MI, a posterolateral MR jet can occur due to tented posterior leaflet or flail anterior leaflet. In this patient with inferior MI the likely mechanism of MR is posterolateral displacement of papillary muscle causing apical tethering of posterior mitral leaflet, especially P2 and P3 segments. This jet would be posteriorly directed and originates at the medial commissure.

107. **Answer: A.**

In the presence of severe AR, the pressure half-time is decreased due to a rise in LV diastolic pressure produced by AR. Hence in the calculation of mitral valve area by the pressure half-time method the valve area will be overestimated or mitral stenosis severity will be underestimated. Pressure half-time is decreased due to increase in late left ventricular diastolic pressure, causing a reduction in the LA–LV gradient.

108. **Answer: A.**

ASD will cause left atrial decompression, and hence would result in rapid reduction in the LA–LV diastolic gradient through diastole, decreasing the pressure half-time. This will cause overestimation of the mitral valve area.

109. **Answer: A.**

The peak inflow rate has to be corrected for the inlet angle as the shape of the PISA is not hemispheric, but two-thirds of a hemisphere. Hence the peak flow rate is given by the formula $2 \times 3.14 \times r^2 \times$ angle of inlet/180 × aliasing velocity. By this formula the flow rate divided by the peak inflow velocity in cm/s gives the mitral valve area in cm^2.

110. **Answer: C.**

The transmitral flow volume per beat would be the same as the stroke volume, i.e. 70 cc/beat. In the absence of MR, the effective diastolic mitral orifice area would be $70 \, cc/50 = 1.4 \, cm^2$.

111. **Answer: B.**

The effective regurgitant volume is $42 \, cm^3$ (112 − 70). The ERO area is the effective regurgitant volume (cm^3)/TVI of MR signal (cm). Hence, $42/60 = 0.7 \, cm^2$. The ERO area is $0.7 \, cm^2$. Please note the units of each of the measurements: in addition, the flow rate is in cm^3/s. Paying attention to these is helpful in formulating the various equations. For example the ERO area can also be obtained by dividing the peak regurgitant flow rate obtained by the PISA method (which is in cm^3/s) by the peak regurgitant velocity (which is in cm/s) such that the unit of measurement remains in cm^2.

112. **Answer. A.**

The true forward stroke volume is 75 cc/beat in the absence of pulmonary regurgitation. Mitral regurgitant volume is $120 − 75 = 45$ cc and aortic regurgitant volume is $90 − 75 = 15$ cc. Dividing the regurgitant volume by their respective TVIs will yield their effective regurgitant orifice area.

113. **Answer. C.**

Regurgitant volume is $140 − 80 = 60$ cc/beat and regurgitant fraction is $60/140 = 44\%$. Effective regurgitant orifice area is regurgitant volume/TVI of aortic signal, i.e. $60/100 = 0.6 \, cm^2$. The regurgitant fraction in AR depends not only on ERO, but diastolic period and driving pressure. Hence the ERO area is a more reliable index of AR volumetric severity. An ERO area of $\geq 0.4 \, cm^2$ is indicative of severe AR.

114. **Answer: B.**

End-diastolic PR velocity of 2 m/s represents a PA–RV end diastolic gradient of 16 mmHg. Assuming an RV end diastolic pressure of 10 mmHg (same as RA pressure), the PA diastolic pressure will be 26 mmHg, which is in the moderate range.

115. **Answer: B.**

Systolic gradient across the pulmonary valve does not affect the diastolic pressure gradient based on the simplified Bernoulli equation. The only two determinants of

PA end diastolic pressure are the PA–RV end diastolic gradient and the RV end diastolic pressure, which is assumed to be equal to the RA pressure.

116. **Answer: C.**

In this patient RV end diastolic pressure equals RA pressure – tricuspid stenosis diastolic gradient ($10 - 8 = 2$ mmHg). The PA end diastolic pressure will be $16 + 2 = 18$ mmHg.

117. **Answer: A.**

In this patient, the estimated right ventricular systolic pressure (RVSP) is $64 + 6$ mmHg $= 70$ mmHg. Pressure drop across the pulmonary valve is equal to 25 mmHg, resulting in a systolic pressure of 45 mmHg in the main PA. As there is 3–4 cm between the pulmonary valve and the right PA, flow streams would have normalized and would allow us to estimate the pressure drop at the branch stenosis without the limitations of stenosis in series unless there is a substantial pressure recovery. As the pressure drop across the branch stenosis is 25 mmHg, estimated systolic pressure distal to the branch stenosis is $45 - 25$ or 20 mmHg.

118. **Answer: A.**

The RV systolic pressure is 110 mmHg based on TR velocity ($5 \times 5 \times 4 + 10 = 110$ mmHg). VSD peak velocity is 3 m/s corresponding to an LV–RV pressure gradient of 36 mmHg. Given the systemic systolic pressure of 146 mmHg (hence an LV systolic pressure of 146 mmHg), the VSD gradient is again concordant with an RV systolic pressure of 110 mmHg. In the absence of PS, this is the pressure in the proximal PA. The pressure gradient across the band is $4.7 \times 4.7 \times 4 = 88$ mmHg. Hence the PA systolic pressure distal to the band is $110 - 88 = 22$ mmHg. Though technically this patient has severe elevation of proximal PA pressure, the PA vascular perfusion pressure is normal, indicating the absence of pulmonary artery disease, making this patient a candidate for surgical closure of VSD.

119. **Answer: A.**

The stroke volume equals the cross-sectional area $\times$ TVI of LVOT, which is $3.14 \times 1 \times 1 \times 25 = 78$ cc. Stroke volume multiplied by heart rate, i.e. $78 \times 70 = 5.5$ L/min, equals cardiac output.

120. **Answer: D.**

In a patient with serial stenosis in close proximity, the continuity equation cannot be applied because of difficulty in obtaining precise subvalvular velocity and cross-sectional area of the flow in the LVOT. In a person without systolic anterior motion the cross-sectional area of subvalvular flow is roughly equal to the cross-sectional area of the LV outflow tract. Subvalvular obstruction will result in flow streams such that the cross-sectional area of flow is less than the anatomic LVOT area.

Chapter 7

121. Bicuspid aortic valve may be associated with:
    A. Coronary anomalies
    B. Coarctation of the aorta
    C. Atrial septal defect
    D. None of the above

122. A dilated coronary sinus could be seen in all of the following conditions except:
    A. Right atrial hypertension
    B. Persistent left superior vena cava
    C. Coronary A–V fistula
    D. Unroofed coronary sinus
    E. Azygos continuity of inferior vena cava

123. Atrial septal defect (ASD) of sinus venosus type is most commonly associated with:
    A. Anomalous drainage of right upper pulmonary vein into right atrium
    B. Anomalous drainage of left upper pulmonary vein into right atrium
    C. Persistent left upper superior vena cava
    D. Coronary artery anomalies

124. Ostium primum ASD is most commonly associated with:
    A. Cleft anterior mitral leaflet
    B. Cleft in septal leaflet of tricuspid valve
    C. Patent ductus arteriosus
    D. Aortic stenosis

125. Dilatation of the pulmonary artery is seen in all of the following conditions except:
    A. Atrial septal defect
    B. Valvular pulmonary stenosis
    C. Infundibular pulmonary stenosis
    D. Pulmonary hypertension

126. Risk of aortic dissection is increased in the following conditions except:
    A. Marfan's syndrome
    B. Bicuspid aortic valve
    C. Pregnancy
    D. Mitral stenosis

127. A 52-year-old patient with a 31 mm St. Jude mitral valve has severe shortness of breath. Left ventricular function and aortic valve are normal. The disc motion of the prosthetic

valve is normal. Analysis of transmitral flow with continuous wave Doppler revealed an E-wave velocity of 2.6 m/s, A-wave velocity of 0.6 m/s, E-wave pressure half-time 40 ms, diastolic mean gradient of 6 mmHg at a heart rate of 60/min, isovolumic relaxation time (IVRT) 30 ms. This patient is likely to have:

A. Mitral regurgitation

B. Pannus growth into the prosthetic valve

C. Prosthetic valve thrombosis

D. Normal prosthetic valve function

128. In a person with suspected paravalvular (mechanical) mitral regurgitation, the following transducer position has the best chance of revealing the mitral regurgitation jet:

A. Parasternal long axis view

B. Apical four-chamber

C. Apical two-chamber

D. Apical long axis

129. A patient with a bileaflet mechanical aortic valve has shortness of breath on exertion. An echocardiogram revealed normal left ventricular systolic function and mitral valve function. The left ventricular outflow tract (LVOT) dimension was 2.2 cm, LVOT (V_1) velocity was 1.5 m/s and aortic transvalvular velocity (V_2) was 4.5 m/s, with no aortic regurgitation. Measurements obtained 2 years earlier when the patient was asymptomatic were: LVOT diameter 2.2 cm, V_1 0.9 m/s and V_2 2.7 m/s. Likely cause of this patient's shortness of breath is:

A. Prosthetic valve stenosis

B. Patient–prosthesis mismatch

C. High cardiac output state, patient may be anemic

D. None of the above

130. A patient with a mechanical prosthetic mitral valve has gastrointestinal bleeding and the following measurements were obtained: diastolic mean gradient 11 mmHg, peak gradient 16 mmHg, pressure half-time 65 ms, heart rate 114/min. This increased gradient is likely to be:

A. Normal

B. Abnormal

C. Cannot comment

131. The following measurements were obtained in a patient with mitral regurgitation: proximal isovelocity surface area (PISA) radius 1 cm at a Nyquist limit of 50 cm/s, peak mitral regurgitation velocity 5 m/sec and mitral regurgitation signal time velocity integral 100 cm. The regurgitant volume is:

A. 63 cc/beat

B. 31 cc/beat

C. 63 cc/s

D. 63%

132. Distribution of leaflet thickening and calcification in rheumatic mitral stenosis is:

A. More at the tip

B. More at the base

C. Uniform throughout the leaflets

133. Leaflet calcification in degenerative mitral stenosis is:
    A. More at the tip
    B. More at the base
    C. Uniform throughout the leaflets

134. The predominant mechanism of chronic ischemic mitral regurgitation is:
    A. Restriction of mitral leaflet closure
    B. Papillary muscle dysfunction
    C. Ruptured chordae tendinae
    D. Ruptured papillary muscle

135. In a person with chronic ischemic mitral regurgitation (MR) due to old inferior myocardial infarction (MI) and an ejection fraction of 50%, the location of the MR jet would be:
    A. Medial commissure
    B. Lateral Commissure
    C. Central

136. In the above patient the jet direction would be:
    A. Posterior
    B. Anterior
    C. Central

137. In a patient with old anteroseptal MI with an ejection fraction of 28%, an ischemic MR jet is likely to be:
    A. Central
    B. Lateral wall hugging
    C. Medial wall hugging

138. Mitral regurgitation in aortic stenosis is related to which of these factors:
    A. Degree of mitral annular calcification
    B. Severity of aortic stenosis
    C. An increase in LV end systolic dimension
    D. Degree of aortic leaflet calcification

139. Left atrial myxoma may be differentiated from a left atrial thrombus by all of the following characteristics except:
    A. Enhancement with transpulmonary contrast agent
    B. Presence of blood vessels on color flow imaging
    C. Attachment to the atrial septum
    D. Similar mass in the left ventricle (LV) with normal LV function.

140. The most common location of left atrial thrombus is:
    A. Left atrial appendage
    B. Body
    C. Atrial septum
    D. Atrial roof

Answers for chapter 7

121. **Answer: B.**

Bicuspid valve is associated with coarctation of the aorta. Biscuspid aortic valve occurs in 1–2% of the population. In these people aortic coarctation is rare, but 25% of patients with coarctation have a bicuspid aortic valve.

122. **Answer: E.**

Coronary sinus can be dilated due to increased pressure or flow. There is increased flow in the coronary sinus in the left superior vena cava, which drains into the coronary sinus, coronary A–V fistula due to increased shunt, and unroofed coronary sinus due to increased flow from left atrium (LA) to coronary sinus. Right atrial hypertension causes increased pressure, which will lead to dilated coronary sinus.

123. **Answer: A.**

ASD of sinus venosus type is most commonly associated with anomalous drainage of the right upper pulmonary vein into the right atrium.

124. **Answer: A.**

Ostium primum ASD is most commonly associated with a cleft anterior mitral leaflet. This is a form of endocardial cushion defect.

125. **Answer: C.**

Infundibular pulmonary stenosis is not associated with dilatation of the pulmonary artery. Poststenotic dilatation is seen only in valvular pulmonary stenosis and not in subvalvular pulmonary stenosis. In ASD the pulmonary artery dilates due to increased flow and in pulmonary hypertension dilatation is due to increased pressure. Idiopathic dilatation of the pulmonary artery can also occur. Marfan syndrome is a cause of pulmonary artery dilatation as well.

126. **Answer: D.**

All conditions except mitral stenosis have weakened media predisposing to dissection. Hypertension can also increase the risk for dissection.

127. **Answer: A.**

Normal IVRT is 70–100 ms, and pressure half-time is 65–80 ms for a prosthetic mitral valve. With a normal cardiac output the mean gradient would be 3–4 mmHg at a heart rate of 60/min. Shortened IVRT, short pressure half-time and high E/A ratio indicate high LA pressure. A stenotic prosthetic valve would have caused increase in pressure half-time and an increase in mean gradient far more than 6 mmHg at a heart rate of 60/min. A mildly increased gradient despite a shortened pressure half-time indicates increased transvalvular flow suggestive of mitral regurgitation, which may be difficult to visualize from a transthoracic echo. Hence a transesophageal echocardiogram (TEE) would be warranted. High LA pressure without an increase in flow would result in shortened IVRT and pressure half-time without an increase in the gradient. A good example of this is superadded restrictive cardiomyopathy.

128. **Answer: A.**

Shadowing in the left atrium is least with a parasternal long axis view, however TEE is the best technique to evaluate for paravalvular mitral leaks.

129. **Answer: C.**

An unchanged V_1/V_2 ratio compared to prior echo confirms the absence of prosthetic valve stenosis. An elevated V_1 indicates elevated cardiac output and the transvalvular gradient is flow dependent. Anemia is a common problem secondary to blood loss due to anticoagulation, and less commonly due to mechanical hemolysis. Patient prosthesis mismatch occurs when the valve is too small for the cardiac output needs of the patient. The effective aortic orifice area in this patient is about 1.3 cm². There is no change in the intrinsic valvular function in this patient.

130. **Answer: A.**

The measurements are normal. Pressure half-time of 65 ms indicates normal valve function. Mean gradient is appropriately increased due to tachycardia (which shortens the diastolic filling period), anemia and possibly high cardiac output. Prosthetic valves are intrinsically mildly stenotic.

131. **Answer: A.**

Effective regurgitant orifice area is given by the formula $2\pi r^2 \times$ Nyquist limit / MR velocity, i.e. $2 \times 3.14 \times 1 \times 1 \times 50 / 500$ cm/s $= 0.628$ cm². Regurgitant volume is effective regurgitant orifice area (in cm²) × TVI (in cm). In this patient it is $0.628 \times 100 = 62.8$ cc. This is per beat and not per second.

132. **Answer: A.**

133. **Answer: B.**

Calcification extends from the annulus, i.e in a centripetal fashion compared to rheumatic, which is centrifugal.

134. **Answer: A.**

Restriction, tethering and tenting refer to the phenomenon of incomplete systolic closure due to apical traction on the mitral leaflets due to outward displacement of the papillary muscles. This causes tenting of the leaflets and the coaptation point is displaced apically. This is not due to contractile failure of the papillary muscles (papillary muscle dysfunction). Papillary muscle rupture causes acute MR, leading to pulmonary edema and hemodynamic compromise.

135. **Answer: A.**

Due to displacement of the posteromedial papillary muscle, there is tethering of medial portions of both leaflet (P3 and A3) segments causing a medial commissural jet. When the left ventricle (LV) is uniformly dilated, the jet could be central in origin.

136. **Answer: B.**

As there is greater tenting of P3 than A3, the jet is directed posteriorly. There may also be some tenting of P2.

137. **Answer: A.**

In an anterior MI, there is generally remodeling of the noninfarcted segments as well, causing dilatation of the whole LV cavity. This is reflected by a low ejection fraction. This causes displacement of both papillary muscles and tenting of all segments of both leaflets, giving rise to central MR, although exceptions may occur. MR in dilated cardiomyopathy occurs because of a similar mechanism.

138. **Answer: C.**

The mechanism of MR is functional and is related to LV dilation and leaflet tethering. Aortic leaflet calcification, mitral annular calcification and severity of aortic stenosis contribute very little in the genesis of MR. A higher driving pressure in more severe degrees of aortic stenosis may increase the regurgitant volume and the jet area, but will not cause MR in the absence of a defect in the mitral coaptation mechanism.

139. **Answer: C.**

Myxomas are vascular: blood vessels may be seen on color flow imaging and enhanced mildly with transpulmonary contrast agent. Though left atrial thrombus is most commonly seen in the appendage, it may be attached to the atrial septum or may traverse through a patent foramen ovale from the right side (paradoxical embolism). The presence of a mass in the LV in the face of normal LV function makes a thrombus unlikely and points to a familial myxoma syndrome (Carney's syndrome).

140. **Answer: A.**

This generally occurs in the presence of atrial fibrillation or flutter. The probability is increased by the presence of mitral stenosis, heart failure, low ejection fraction, large left atrium and left atrial spontaneous echo contrast.

Chapter 8

141. The most common benign tumor in the heart is:
    A. Left atrial myxoma
    B. Papillary fibroelastoma
    C. Lamble's excrescences
    D. Fibroma

142. The most common metastatic malignant tumor of the heart is:
    A. Melanoma
    B. Fibrosarcoma
    C. Rhabdomyoma
    D. Liposarcoma

143. In a person with flail P2 segment of the posterior mitral leaflet (PML), the mitral regurgitation (MR) jet is likely to be:
    A. Posterior wall hugging
    B. Anterior wall hugging
    C. Central
    D. Cannot comment

144. In a person with flail A2 segment of the anterior mitral leaflet (AML), the MR jet is likely to be:
    A. Posterior wall hugging
    B. Anterior wall hugging
    C. Central
    D. Cannot comment

145. Total surface area of mitral leaflets is generally ———% of mitral annular area.
    A. 100%
    B. 120%
    C. 150%
    D. 200%

146. The PML compared to the AML is:
    A. Shorter
    B. Longer
    C. Same length as the anterior leaflet
    D. Of variable length

147. The length of the posterior leaflet attachment to the mitral annulus compared to that of the AML is:
    A. Shorter
    B. Longer
    C. Same
    D. Variable

148. In an apical long-axis view the following mitral leaflet segments are seen:
    A. A2P2
    B. A3P3
    C. A1P1
    D. A3P1

149. Apical two-chamber view is likely to show the following mitral leaflet segments:
    A. P1A2P3
    B. A2P2
    C. A3P1
    D. A1P1

150. The major diameter of the mitral annulus is best imaged from:
    A. Apical two-chamber view
    B. Apical long axis view
    C. Apical five-chamber view
    D. Parasternal long axis view

151. The MR jet is best visualized in parasternal long axis view when the transducer tip is directed more inferomedially. The location of the MR jet in this patient is:
    A. Medial commissure
    B. Lateral commissure
    C. Central

152. A continuous flow is visualized in the main pulmonary artery. This could be related to:
    A. Patent ductus arteriosus (PDA)
    B. Coronary A–V fistula
    C. Idiopathic dilatation of main pulmonary artery
    D. None of the above

153. Echocardiographic features of anatomic right ventricle in a congenitally corrected transposition of great vessels are all of the following except:
    A. Trileaflet A–V valve
    B. Apical position of associated A–V valve
    C. Presence of moderator band
    D. Wall thickness <7 mm

154. Problems encountered with congenitally corrected great arteries are all of the following except:
    A. Failure of systemic ventricle
    B. Tricuspid regurgitation

C. Atrial and ventricular arrhythmias

D. Aortic regurgitation

155. Features of Tetralogy of Fallot are all of the following except:
    A. Overriding aorta
    B. Nonrestrictive ventricular septal defect (VSD)
    C. Pulmonary stenosis
    D. Right ventricular (RV) hypertrophy
    E. Atrial septal defect (ASD)

156. Associations of atrial septal aneurysm include all of the following except:
    A. Patent foramen ovale
    B. Atrial arrythmias
    C. Transient ischemic attacks
    D. Pulmonary hypertension

157. Echocardiographic findings in Ebstein's anomaly may include:
    A. Apical displacement of the septal leaflet of the tricuspid valve > 8 mm compared to position of AML attachment
    B. Large, septal tricuspid leaflet with tethering to RV wall
    C. Tricuspid regurgitation
    D. Atrial septal defect
    E. Hypoplastic pulmonary arteries

158. The most common location of the accessory pathway in Ebstein's anomaly is:
    A. Posteroseptal
    B. Anteroseptal
    C. Right lateral
    D. Left lateral

159. The following type of ventricular septal defect is likely to be associated with aortic regurgitation:
    A. Perimembranous
    B. Muscular
    C. Supracristal
    D. Inlet

160. In a patient with secundum ASD, the following features are consistent with amenability of percutaneous closure except:
    A. Defect size of 22 mm
    B. Mitral rim of 8 mm
    C. Aortic rim of 2 mm
    D. Inferior vena cava rim of 1 mm

Answers for chapter 8

141. **Answer: B.**
Papillary fibroelastoma is the most common benign tumor seen in the heart, followed by myxoma.

142. **Answer: A.**
The most common metastatic malignancy of the heart is melanoma, followed by lung and breast cancer. Primary malignant tumors of the heart are rare, but rhabdomyoma is the commonest.

143. **Answer: B.**
The jet is away from the flail segment in contrast to a tethered segment.

144. **Answer: A.**

145. **Answer: C.**
Normally there is 50% more leaflet tissue than annular area to cause a 2–3 mm leaflet overlap at the coaptation margin. The absolute leaflet area is increased in myxomatous mitral valve disease and hypertrophic cardiomyopathy. The normal annular area is roughly 7–8 cm^2 and the leaflet area is 10–12 cm^2.

146. **Answer: A.**
The posterior leaflet length is 10–14 mm and the anterior leaflet length is 20–24 mm.

147. **Answer: B.**
This results in equal surface area of anterior and posterior leaflets.

148. **Answer: A.**
This view cuts through the middle of both leaflets, i.e. A2 and P2.

149. **Answer: A.**
Two-chamber view goes through the intercommissural plane and cuts through P1 and P3, with A2 seen between them in systole. A medial tilt of the transducer will cut the AML entirely showing A1A2A3, and a lateral tilt will cut the PML entirely revealing P1P2P3.

150. **Answer: A.**
Equivalent to this on a TEE examination is the mid-esophageal view at 70–80°. Apical long axis view gives the minor dimension of the mitral annulus.

151. **Answer: A.**
Tilting the transducer from this location towards the left shoulder will reveal the lateral commissure.

152. **Answer: A.**
The PDA drains at the origin of the left pulmonary artery. Anomalous origin of coronary artery from pulmonary artery can cause continuous flow because of retrograde flow into the pulmonary artery. Both are examples of left to right shunts. Dilatation of the pulmonary artery can cause swirling of blood in the pulmonary artery in systole, giving a false impression of shunt flow because of reversed flow direction.

153. **Answer: D.**

Ventricles go with corresponding A–V valves, i.e. right ventricle with tricuspid valve and left ventricle with mitral valve. Wall thickness is not a reliable feature. In right ventricular hypertrophy the wall thickness may be >7 mm and the pulmonary left ventricle may have a wall thickness of <7 mm.

154. **Answer: D.**

The systemic RV has a high likelihood of failure. It may also have myocardial perfusion defects. Tricuspid valve failure is common secondary to annular dilatation. Atrial and ventricular arrhythmias are common due to dilatation of the left atrium and systemic RV. Presence of atrial arrhythmias may contribute to RV dysfunction.

155. **Answer: E.**

ASD is not a feature in classical Tetralogy of Fallot. Presence of ASD in Tetralogy has been referred to as the Pentalogy of Fallot.

156. **Answer: D.**

The left to right shunt through the patent foramen ovale (PFO) is generally very small and hence pulmonary hypertension is not seen with an aneurysmal atrial septum. Risk of transient ischemic attack is highest when PFO and atrial septal aneurysm coexist and the shunt flow is large. Speculated mechanisms for this include paradoxical embolism, *in situ* thrombus formation and atrial arrhythmias.

157. **Answer: E.**

Hypoplastic pulmonary arteries is not a feature. ASD may co-exist and in the presence of tricuspid regurgitation may result in right to left shunt, causing cyanosis.

158. **Answer: C.**

Right lateral.

159. **Answer: C.**

In this type of VSD there is loss of support to the right coronary cusp of the aortic valve, which will result in aortic regurgitation.

160. **Answer: D.**

The maximum stretched diameter of the defect that can be closed is 40 mm with an Amplatzer device provided that the septum is large enough to allow the 8 mm flange all around, making the total disc diameter on the left atrial side 56 mm. Aortic rim is the least important and not essential. Inadequacy of other rims may result not only in the impingement of the discs on related structures, but device instability and dislodgement. Proximity of superior vena cava rim to right upper pulmonary vein is important as well.

Chapter 9

161. Diagnostic sensitivity of stress echocardiography is higher with:
    A. One-vessel disease
    B. Two-vessel disease
    C. Three-vessel disease
    D. All of the above

162. False-positive rate for stress echocardiography is high for which group of patients:
    A. Low probability of coronary artery disease (CAD)
    B. Intermediate probability of CAD
    C. High probability of CAD
    D. Independent of CAD

163. Negative predictive value of stress echo is lowest in this group of patients:
    A. Low probability of CAD
    B. Intermediate probability of CAD
    C. High probability of CAD
    D. Independent of CAD

164. False-positive wall motion abnormalities are most commonly seen in which of the following myocardial segments?
    A. Posterior basal wall
    B. Anterior septum
    C. Lateral wall
    D. Apex

165. The usual response of left ventricular (LV) end systolic size during exercise is:
    A. Reduction
    B. Increase
    C. Variable response
    D. No change

166. An increase in LV end systolic volume during stress may occur in all of the situations except:
    A. Multivessel CAD
    B. Left main CAD
    C. Hypertensive blood pressure response
    D. Left ventricular hypertrophy

167. A 53-year-old patient is undergoing dobutamine stress echocardiography (DSE). At 20 µg dose the blood pressure drops from 140/80 mmHg to 80/50 mmHg associated with severe nausea, and the heart rate dropped from 110/min to 60/min. The most likely cause of this response is:
    A. Left ventricular cavity obliteration causing a vagal response
    B. Severe ischemic response due to multivessel CAD
    C. 2:1 A–V block produced by ischemia in right coronary artery territory
    D. None of the above

168. What proportion of normal patients undergoing DSE may have a drop in their blood pressure:
    A. Zero
    B. 20%
    C. 50%
    D. 89%

169. All of the following factors affect pulmonary vein A-wave amplitude except:
    A. LV end diastolic stiffness
    B. Left atrial function
    C. Pulmonary vein diameter
    D. Heart rate
    E. Pulmonary artery pressure

170. The pulmonary vein S wave may be less prominent than the D wave in the following situations except:
    A. Young children
    B. Moderate to severe mitral regurgitation
    C. Atrial fibrillation
    D. Elevated left atrial (LA) pressure
    E. Abnormal LV relaxation with normal left atrial (LA) pressure

171. Normal pulmonary vein A-wave duration compared to mitral A-wave duration is:
    A. Less
    B. More
    C. Same
    D. Variable

172. Normal pulmonary vein D-wave deceleration in an adult is:
    A. 50–100 ms
    B. 100–170 ms
    C. 170–260 ms
    D. Highly variable

173. Increased pulmonary vein D-wave deceleration time may be encountered in:
    A. Mitral stenosis
    B. Mitral regurgitation
    C. High LA pressure
    D. Pulmonary stenosis

174. Normal mitral E-wave propagation velocity by color M mode inside the LV is:
    A. 10–30 cm/s
    B. 30–50 cm/sec
    C. Greater than 50 cm/s
    D. Greater than 500 cm/s

175. A reduced mitral E-wave propagation velocity indicates:
    A. High LA pressure
    B. Increased tau
    C. Reduced tau
    D. Increased modulus LV chamber stiffness

176. A reduced A-wave transit time to the LV outflow tract is indicative of:
    A. Low negative dp/dt
    B. Increased tau
    C. Reduced tau
    D. Increased modulus of LV chamber stiffness

177. Rate of acceleration of the early portion of the aortic regurgitation (AR) signal is determined by:
    A. LV negative dp/dt
    B. LV positive dp/dt
    C. LV end diastolic pressure
    D. Aortic end diastolic pressure

178. Rapidly decelerating terminal portion of the AR signal is mainly influenced by:
    A. LV negative dp/dt
    B. LV positive dp/dt
    C. LV end diastolic pressure
    D. Aortic end diastolic pressure

179. A patient has mild mitral regurgitation and the time taken for mitral regurgitation velocity to drop from 3 m/s velocity to 1 m/s on continuous wave Doppler examination was 40 ms. The average rate of LV pressure decay in this patient is:
    A. 3600 mmHg/s
    B. 1280 mm/s
    C. 800 mm/s
    D. 400 mm/s

180. By tissue velocity imaging, the mitral annular Sm wave is produced by:
    A. Annular descent during systole
    B. Annular ascent during systole
    C. Atrial contraction
    D. LV relaxation

Answers for chapter 9

161. **Answer: C.**

    It is about 50% for one-vessel disease and 80% for three-vessel disease.

162. **Answer: A.**

    Based on Baye's theorem, the diagnostic accuracy is highest for intermediate probability, and in patients with extremely low probability most of the tests will be false positive, yielding a low positive predictive value. Positive predictive value (PPV) is the proportion of patients with positive tests who truly have disease. In other words, $PPV = TP/(TP + FP)$.

163. **Answer: C.**

    Testing this group of patients is likely to yield a high proportion of patients with a false-negative test, hence lowering the negative predictive value (NPV). In other words, $NPV = TN/TN + FN$.

164. **Answer: A.**

    Wall motion abnormality in the posterior basal wall is most difficult to analyze due to a range of normalcy, proximity to valvular plane and the apical displacement of the wall during systole, which results in imaging of different parts of the inferior wall during systole and diastole in the short axis view. False positivity during stress echocardiography is in the range of 40–50% for this wall.

165. **Answer: A.**

    Reduction due to a combination of reduced systemic vascular resistance (SVR) and increased LV contractility.

166. **Answer: D.**

    This is the equivalent of transient ischemic dilatation of the LV on stress nuclear perfusion imaging.

167. **Answer: A.**

    This is typical of a vasovagal response that is preceded by a hyperdynamic response, which triggers this. This may be exaggerated by volume depletion and may potentially be prevented by volume loading. When a hyperdynamic response with cavity obliteration is seen, instead of increasing the dobutamine dose, atropine should be administered to increase the heart rate. This will help to avert a vagal response. Drop in SVR is universal during DSE and may not be fully compensated by cardiac output increase. Systolic anterior movement can occur during DSE, especially in patients with LV hypotension who develop a hyperdynamic response, but LV outflow tract obstruction is rarely responsible for hypotension. Hypotension in such patients, when it occurs, is generally due to a vagal response produced by the hyperdynamic LV stimulating the vagal C type of fibers in the LV wall. This response could be partially prevented by volume loading before DSE.

168. **Answer: B.**

    Drop in blood pressure during DSE does not have the same clinical significance as in a regular exercise stress test. This is because normal cardiac output increase during

DSE is only 50–80%, which is far less than exercise. Dobutamine causes peripheral vasodilatation.

169. **Answer: E.**

The amplitude is increased in the presence of a stiff LV and reduced in left atrial mechanical failure. The pulmonary A wave may disappear with heart rates in excess of 100/min, where flow may be entirely antegrade, and atrial contraction may produce a transient deceleration pulmonary flow without reversal. As velocity depends upon flow volume and cross-sectional area, a dilated pulmonary vein is likely to reduce the A-wave velocity and a collapsed vein in a dry patient can result in a giant A wave.

170. **Answer: E.**

Young children have very efficient LV relaxation properties, resulting in rapid early filling (mitral E wave) paralleled by an increase in D wave that might have rapid deceleration as well. As S1 is due to atrial relaxation, atrial fibrillation results in reduced S-wave amplitude. Systolic left atrial filling from mitral regurgitation will impede pulmonary vein flow in systole. High LA pressure renders the LA less compliant due to rightward shift of its pressure–volume curve and hence will impede atrial systolic filling, as LA is a closed chamber receiving only pulmonary venous flow during systole. Abnormal LV relaxation reduces E- and D-wave amplitudes, resulting in an increase in S-wave amplitude in the absence of elevated LA pressure.

171. **Answer: A.**

Increased pulmonary A-wave duration compared to mitral A-wave duration indicates high LV end diastolic pressure. Delta duration of more than 30 ms is very suggestive of high LV end diastolic pressure.

172. **Answer: C.**

Reduced D-wave deceleration time indicates high LA pressure very similar to mitral E-wave deceleration time.

173. **Answer: A.**

The D-wave deceleration time parallels mitral E-wave deceleration time and the slope is flatter in mitral stenosis. It may also be prolonged in patients with prosthetic mitral valves and abnormal LV relaxation. The deceleration time is reduced with high left atrial pressure. Pulmonary stenosis has no known effect on this slope.

174. **Answer: C.**

Greater than 50 cm/s.

175. **Answer: B.**

Slower propagation indicates abnormal LV relaxation, and this is reflected by increased tau by invasive measurement.

176. **Answer: D.**

The A-wave propagation is an end diastolic phenomenon and its propagation velocity is increased with increased LV end diastolic stiffness. Increased propagation velocity results in a shorter transit time. The modulus of chamber stiffness is a measure of operative LV stiffness.

177. **Answer: A.**

     Assuming a constant aortic pressure during this short time, rate of acceleration is principally determined by LV pressure decay after aortic valve closure during the LV isovolumic relaxation period. For example, at the 1 m/s point the aortic–LV pressure gradient is 4 mmHg and at 2.5 m/s it is 25 mmHg. Assuming a constant aortic pressure, the drop in LV pressure between these two points is $25 - 4 = 21$ mmHg. The rate of LV pressure drop would be 21/time taken for AR signal to increase from 1 m/s to 2.5 m/s. For example, if this time interval is 20 ms (0.02 s) the average negative LV dp/dt would be $21/0.02 = 1050$ mmHg/s.

178. **Answer: B.**

     This rapidly decelerating terminal portion of AR occurs during the isovolumic contraction period and the LV positive dp/dt may be calculated with similar assumptions as for the LV negative dp/dt between 2.5 m/s and 1 m/s points of the AR signal.

179. **Answer: C.**

     The LV negative $dp/dt = 36 - 4/0.04 = 800$ mmHg/s. This again assumes a constant LA pressure during this portion of LV isovolumic contraction time. This noninvasive measure has been validated against invasively derived negative dp/dt by high-fidelity LV pressure recordings.

180. **Answer: A.**

     Annular descent produced by LV long axis shortening causes a positive systolic deflection recorded from the apical view.

Chapter 10

181. Compared to timing of mitral E-wave peak, mitral annular Em peak is:
    A. Earlier
    B. Later
    C. Simultaneous
    D. No relationship

182. Post-ejection left ventricular (LV) shortening may be found in all of the following conditions except:
    A. Hypertensive heart disease
    B. Ischemic cardiomyopathy
    C. Cardiac syndrome X
    D. Mitral stenosis

183. Compared to the epicardial, endocardial radial velocities are:
    A. Higher
    B. Lower
    C. Similar
    D. Variable

184. The following myocardial velocities were obtained from the posterior wall by color Doppler tissue imaging: peak systolic epicardial velocity 2 cm/s, peak systolic endocardial velocity 16 cm/s, systolic LV wall thickness 1.4 cm, early diastolic epicardial velocity 3 cm/s, endocardial velocity 18 cm/s and diastolic wall thickness 1 cm. The systolic transmural velocity gradient in this patient is:
    A. 10/s
    B. 14 cm/s
    C. 19.6 cm/s
    D. 19.6/s

185. For the patient in question 184, diastolic myocardial velocity gradient for the posterior wall is:
    A. 15/s
    B. 1.5/s
    C. 18/s
    D. 18 cm/s

186. In a person with cardiomyopathy, the following Doppler measurements were obtained: Q wave to aortic flow 140 ms, Q wave to pulmonary flow 70 ms, Q to medial mitral

annular Sm wave 70 ms, Q to anterior mitral annular Sm wave 85 ms, Q to lateral Sm wave 140 ms and Q to posterior wall Sm wave 130 ms. Interventricular asynchrony in this patient is:

A. 70 ms
B. 140 ms
C. 85 ms
D. 50 ms

187. In the patient in question 186, LV intraventricular asynchrony is:

A. 70 ms
B. 140 ms
C. 85 ms
D. 130 ms

188. Stroke risk in a patient with patent foramen ovale (PFO) is influenced by:

A. Size of PFO
B. Atrial septal aneurysm
C. History of prior stroke or transient ischemic attack
D. All of the above
E. None of the above

189. Atrial septal aneurysm may be associated with:

A. Patent foramen ovale
B. Atrial arrythmias
C. Increased stroke risk
D. All of the above
E. None of the above

190. Observational data on percutaneous PFO closure indicate that the benefit is greater with:

A. Larger PFO
B. Complete PFO closure
C. Greater number of previous strokes
D. All of the above
E. None of the above

191. All of the following are probable causes of mitral stenosis except:

A. Rheumatic fever
B. Excessive calcification of the mitral annulus
C. Phen-fen valvulopathy
D. Ischemic heart disease

192. Bicuspid aortic valve may be associated with the following except:

A. Aortic root disease
B. Coarctation of the aorta
C. Aortic stenosis or regurgitation
D. Ventricular septal defect

193. Common cause of aortic stenosis in a 50-year-old individual is:

A. Calcific
B. Bicuspid aortic valve
C. Unicuspid aortic valve
D. Rheumatic heart disease

194. Heart failure with normal ejection fraction can occur in the following except:
    A. Hypertrophic cardiomyopathy
    B. Cardiac amyloid
    C. Restrictive cardiomyopathy
    D. Dilated cardiomyopathy

195. Basic components of a partial AV canal defect include all except:
    A. Inlet ventricular septal defect
    B. Septum primum atrial septal defect
    C. Cleft mitral valve
    D. Widened antero-septal tricuspid commisure

196. Signs of acute aortic regurgitation include:
    A. Premature mitral valve closure
    B. Hyperdynamic LV function
    C. Normal left ventricle size
    D. All of the above
    E. None of the above

197. The following are indicative of severe mitral regurgitation except:
    A. Systolic flow reversal in the pulmonary veins
    B. Regurgitant fraction of >60%
    C. Effective regurgitant orifice area of $\geq 0.4\,cm^2$
    D. Vena contracta diameter of $\leq 0.6\,cm$

198. The following are signs of chronic severe aortic regurgitation except:
    A. Regurgitant fraction $\geq 60\%$
    B. Regurgitant volume of $\geq 60\,cc$
    C. Effective regurgitation orifice area $\leq 0.3\,cm^2$
    D. Vena contracta width $\geq 0.6\,cm$

199. Prosthetic valve gradients are increased in following conditions except:
    A. Anemia
    B. Febrile state
    C. Hypothyroidism
    D. Hyperthyroidism

200. What is the velocity of circumferential fiber shortening (VCF) in a patient with the following measurements: LV end diastolic dimension 50 mm, end systolic dimension 33 mm, LV ejection time 300 ms.
    A. 1.1
    B. 0.9
    C. 34
    D. Cannot be calculated

Answers for chapter 10

181. **Answer: A.**

The Em peak precedes the mitral E peak. This Early LV lengthening is due to a combination of LV recoil and relaxation, which generates the mitral E wave. In patients with abnormal LV relaxation the Em peak may follow the E-wave peak.

182. **Answer: D.**

Post-ejection LV shortening is the phenomenon of continued myocardial segmental contraction even after the end of ejection. This asynchrony of the ending of LV contraction may result in impaired LV pressure decay and hence impaired LV filling.

183. **Answer: A.**

This results in a myocardial velocity gradient. A transmural myocardial velocity gradient is a better index of contractile function compared to endocardial myocardial velocities alone. The myocardial velocity gradient is obtained as (endocardial velocity−epicardial velocity)/wall thickness and reflects the rate of LV wall thickening.

184. **Answer: A.**

Systolic myocardial velocity gradient $= (16-2)/1.4 = 10/s$.

185. **Answer: A.**

Diastolic myocardial velocity gradient $= (18-3)/1 = 15/s$.

186. **Answer: A.**

Interventricular asynchrony is the difference between the time difference in the onset of mechanical systolies of right and left ventricles, generally measured as the time difference in right ventricular (RV) and LV ejection from the corresponding flows at pulmonary and aortic valves. In this patient the electromechanical delay for the RV was 70 ms and for the LV was 140 ms. The difference is 70 ms, which corresponds to interventricular asynchrony.

187. **Answer: A.**

The largest difference between electromechanical delays in the LV is a measure of intraventricular mechanical asynchrony. In this patient $140 - 70 = 70$ ms corresponds to intraventricular asynchrony. Greater than 65 ms is a good predictor for response in terms of reverse remodeling and symptom improvement. As the peak velocities are easier to identify, most of the investigators currently use time to peak velocity rather than time to onset.

188. **Answer: D.**

189. **Answer: D.**

190. **Answer: D.**

191. **Answer: D.**

Ischemic heart disease causes mitral regurgitation but is not a cause of mitral stenosis. All the others can cause mitral stenosis.

192. **Answer: D.**

Ventricular septal defect does not occur as an association with bicuspid aortic valve.

193. **Answer: B.**

The most common cause of aortic stenosis in a 50-yr-old individual in bicuspid aortic valve. Calcific aortic stenosis occurs in individuals older than 70 years. Unicuspid aortic valve occurs in infancy. Rheumatic heart disease occurs children aged 5–15 years, mostly in developing countries.

194. **Answer: D.**

Dilated cardiomyopathy is associated with systolic heart failure. All the others are associated with heart failure and a normal ejection fraction.

195. **Answer: A.**

When inlet VSD is present along with the other defects it constitutes complete AV canal defect. Without the presence of inlet VSD, the other three findings constitute a partial AV canal defect.

196. **Answer: D.**

197. **Answer: D.**

A vena contracta width of ≥ 0.7 cm is suggestive of severe mitral Regurgitation.

198. **Answer: C.**

Effective orifice area in chronic severe aortic regurgitation is $\geq 0.3 \text{cm}^2$. All the other findings are suggestive of severe aortic regurgitation.

199. **Answer: C.**

All the other states except hypothyroidism can cause an increase in prosthetic valve gradients due to increased stroke volume.

200. **Answer: A.**

VCF = fractional shortening/ejection time. In this patient fractional shortening = $50 - 33/50 = 0.34$. Thus VCF is $0.34/0.3 = 1.1$ circumferences/s.

Chapter 11

201. Principal determinants of circumferential wall stress include all of the following except:
    A. Left ventricular (LV) end systolic dimension
    B. Left ventricular (LV) end systolic pressure
    C. Left ventricular (LV) systolic wall thickness
    D. Left ventricular (LV) pressure at mitral valve closure

202. Increase in LV end systolic wall stress is likely to reduce all of the following except:
    A. Ejection fraction
    B. Fractional shortening
    C. Velocity of circumferential shortening
    D. LV positive dp/dt

203. The response of LV end systolic volume to an increase in LV end systolic wall stress would be:
    A. An increase
    B. A decrease
    C. No change

204. In a person with LV dysfunction, compared to a normal individual, a graph showing end systolic wall stress (ESWS) on the x-axis and end systolic volume (ESV) on the y-axis, would be:
    A. Steeper
    B. Flatter
    C. None of the above

205. In response to dobutamine infusion, the ESV–ESWS curve will shift:
    A. Down
    B. Upward
    C. No shift

206. The factor least likely to affect the mitral E/A ratio is:
    A. Tau
    B. Modulus of LV chamber stiffness
    C. Left atrial pressure
    D. LV elastic recoil
    E. Cardioversion for atrial fibrillation performed 2 h ago
    F. Pulmonary artery pressure

207. Factors affecting LV isovolumic relaxation time (IVRT) are all of the following except:
    A. Tau
    B. Left atrial pressure
    C. Heart rate
    D. Moderate aortic regurgitation

208. The factor least likely to diminish mitral A-wave amplitude is:
    A. Recent cardioversion
    B. Myopathic left atrium
    C. An acute rise in LV end diastolic pressure
    D. Severe aortic stenosis with mild LV hypotension and normal LV ejection fraction

209. Both high left atrial (LA) pressure and atrial mechanical failure result in a high E/A ratio. The following is least likely to help in the differential diagnosis in this situation:
    A. E-wave deceleration time
    B. Amplitude and duration of AR wave
    C. Pulmonary vein S/D time velocity integral ratio
    D. Mitral annular velocity with tissue Doppler imaging

210. Which of the changes are least likely to occur in a patient with acute severe aortic regurgitation:
    A. Reduction of A-wave amplitude
    B. Premature presystolic closure of the mitral valve
    C. Diastolic mitral regurgitation
    D. Increased amplitude and duration of pulmonary AR wave
    E. A decrease in mitral Em-wave amplitude

211. A late peaking systolic velocity signal is found in which of the following conditions?
    A. Mitral valve prolapse causing late systolic mitral regurgitation (MR)
    B. MR due to systolic anterior motion of the mitral leaflet
    C. LV cavity obliteration
    D. Acute severe MR

212. The following condition causes a reduction in the acceleration time of pulmonary arterial flow:
    A. Pulmonary stenosis
    B. Pulmonary hypertension
    C. Dilated pulmonary artery
    D. Right ventricular (RV) dysfunction

213. Increased respirophasic variations in transvalvular flows may occur in all of the following conditions except:
    A. Status asthmaticus
    B. Constrictive pericarditis
    C. Cardiac tamponade
    D. A large RV infarct
    E. Hypovolemic shock

214. Intrapericardial pressure is increased in all of the following conditions except:
    A. Cardiac tamponade
    B. Acute massive pulmonary embolism
    C. Acute traumatic rupture of tricuspid valve, causing acute tricuspid regurgitation
    D. Acute RV infarct
    E. Severe aortic stenosis with normal LV function

215. A patient with a St. Jude mitral valve no. 29 has a mean diastolic gradient of 3 mmHg and a pressure half-time of 70 ms at a heart rate of 70 beats/min, This is consistent with:
    A. Normal prosthetic valve function
    B. Prosthetic valve thrombosis
    C. Significant pannus growth
    D. Severe MR

216. A patient with a St. Jude mitral prosthetic valve no. 29 has a mean diastolic gradient of 7 mmHg at a heart rate of 70 beats/min and a pressure half-time of 30 ms. This is consistent with:
    A. Normal prosthetic valve function
    B. Prosthetic valve thrombosis
    C. Significant pannus growth
    D. Severe MR

217. A patient with prosthetic mitral valve no. 29 has a mean diastolic gradient of 10 mmHg at a heart rate of 70 beats /min and a pressure half-time of 200 ms. This is consistent with:
    A. Normal prosthetic valve function
    B. Prosthetic mitral valve stenosis
    C. Severe anemia with high output failure
    D. Severe MR

218. The A2–OS snap interval corresponds to:
    A. Isovolumic relaxation time
    B. Isovolumic contraction time
    C. Pre-ejection period
    D. All of the above

219. In a patient with mitral valve stenosis the A2–OS interval may be shortened by all of the following except:
    A. Severe mitral stenosis
    B. Severe MR
    C. Tachycardia
    D. Abnormal LV relaxation

220. An abnormal LV relaxation pattern is consistent with:
    A. Mean LA pressure of 10 mmHg and LV end diastolic pressure (LVEDP) of 22 mmHg
    B. Mean LA pressure of 22 mmHg and LVEDP of 10 mmHg
    C. Mean LA pressure of 10 mmHg and LVEDP of 12 mmHg
    D. Mean LA pressure of 28 mmHg and LVEDP of 30 mmHg
    E. Mean LA pressure of 28 mmHg and LVEDP of 40 mmHg

Answers for chapter 11

201. **Answer: D.**

Wall stress is the force that myocardial fibers have to overcome in order to affect circumferential shortening. It is proportional to LV size and intracavity pressure and inversively proportional to wall thickness. There are three types of wall stresses operating on the myocardium. Theses are circumferential, radial and meridional.

202. **Answer: D.**

The first three measures are afterload dependent and positive dp/dt is preload dependent. LV end systolic wall stress (ESWS) is a good measure of afterload whereas LV end diastolic wall stress is a good measure of preload.

203. **Answer: A.**

An increase. ESWS/ESV is a good load-independent measure of LV systolic performance; a decrease suggests reduced performance, as this indicates a larger ESV for a given ESWS.

204. **Answer: A.**

An increment in ESV in response to an increase in ESWS is greater in a person with LV dysfunction, making this relationship steeper. Contractile responses to changes in afterload may also be studied by using ejection fraction or fractional shortening in place of ESV. However the response will be in the opposite direction. Also, noninvasively derived LV end systolic pressure (from cuff pressure and carotid pulse tracing) is a reasonable surrogate for ESWS.

205. **Answer: A.**

Dobutamine brings out the LV contractile reserve, causing a reduction in LV end systolic volume for a given ESWS.

206. **Answer: F.**

Tau is an invasive measure of LV relaxation, impairment of which will reduce the E/A ratio. Modulus of LV chamber stiffness is a measure of LV late diastolic stiffness. This affects the A-wave amplitude. High LA pressure increases the E-wave amplitude. Increased elastic recoil as it occurs in a hypercontractile state increases the E-wave amplitude through a suction effect. Atrial mechanical failure is common after cardioversion for atrial fibrillation and may take 1–20 days for full recovery.

207. **Answer: D.**

Impaired relaxation prolongs IVRT through slowing the LV pressure decay between aortic valve closure and mitral valve opening. High LA pressure and a large LA V wave will result in earlier opening of the mitral valve at a higher pressure. Fast heart rate diminishes IVRT partly through an improvement of LV relaxation.

208. **Answer: D.**

Myopathic atrium and recent cardioversion result in reduced A-wave amplitude due to reduced atrial mechanical function. Acute rise in LVEDP results in an acute increase in atrial afterload, diminishing its ejection function, just like any other pumping chamber. Atrial output with its contraction depends upon its preload, afterload and contractility. In aortic stenosis with LV hypotension due to abnormal relaxation, there is reduced early LV filling and a compensatory increase in contribution from left atrial contraction.

209. **Answer: C.**

High LA pressure results in short IVRT, reduced E-wave deceleration time and an increase in pulmonary vein AR-wave duration and amplitude. Mitral E/mitral annular Em ratio is a good indicator of LA pressure. Atrial mechanical failure results in diminution of pulmonary AR reversal and absence of atrial relaxation, which causes a left atrial suction effect and will result in diminution of S-wave amplitude. The S-wave amplitude is diminished in high LA pressure due to increased LA operating stiffness during LV systole, when there is no LA emptying.

210. **Answer: E.**

Acute atrial regurgitation causes a rapid increase in LV end diastolic pressure, diminishing A-wave amplitude or eliminating it due to acutely increased atrial afterload. This may also prematurely close the mitral valve. Atrial contraction on a closed mitral valve will result in exaggerated flow reversal in the pulmonary vein during atrial contraction. None of these phenomena directly affect early diastolic LV mechanics, LV relaxation or early diastolic LV lengthening (Em wave).

211. **Answer: C.**

Causes flow acceleration in late systole due to a severe reduction in flow area that occurs in end systole. Though in mitral valve prolapse and hypertrophic obstructive cardiomyopathy the regurgitant volume may be more towards end systole, the shape of the signal is dictated only by the LV–LA pressure gradient and not by the volume of MR. The LV–LA pressure gradient tends to be maximum in early to mid-systole. In acute severe MR a large V wave causes late systolic deceleration of the signal, a so-called "V wave cut-off sign".

212. **Answer: B.**

This is thought to be due to faster return of the reflected pressure waves because of increased operative stiffness of the pulmonary arterial tree, which causes early deceleration of the flow.

213. **Answer: E.**

In status asthmaticus, exaggerated respiratory variation in intrapleural pressures causes marked variation in venous returns both to the right and left heart during the respiratory cycle. In constriction and tamponade, there is exaggerated interventricular interaction due to septal shifts during respiration, causing an exaggeration of normal flow variations across the valves during the respiratory cycle. RV infarct causes acute RV dilation and invokes pericardial constraint and physiology similar to constrictive pericarditis.

214. **Answer: E.**

In addition to pericardial fluid accumulation, any phenomenon that acutely increases the intrapericardial volume invokes pericardial constraint and hence elevation of the intrapericardial pressure. Massive pulmonary embolus and RV infarct cause acute RV dilation. Any acute regurgitant lesion causes acute chamber dilation and hence invokes pericardial constraint.

215. **Answer: A.**

Both the mean gradient and pressure half-time are useful in assessing and monitoring prosthetic mitral valve function.

216. **Answer: D.**

Reduced pressure half-time is suggestive of high LA pressure and an increased gradient at a normal heart rate is suggestive of increased flow across the mitral valve; this combination is highly suggestive of mitral regurgitation.

217. **Answer: B.**

Stenotic prosthetic valve hemodynamics is similar to native mitral valve stenosis. An increase in gradient is accompanied by an increase in pressure half-time, indicating reduced effective orifice area. High output causes an increase in gradient with a normal or reduced pressure half-time depending upon left atrial pressure.

218. **Answer: A.**

IVRT is the interval between the aortic component of the second heart sound and mitral valve opening.

219. **Answer: D.**

High left atrial pressure that occurs in mitral stenosis or MR will cause earlier opening of the mitral valve, thus causing a shortening of the A2–OS interval. Tachycardia improves LV relaxation and shortens this interval. Abnormal LV relaxation, by reducing the rate of pressure decay between aortic valve closure and mitral valve opening, would lengthen this interval.

220. **Answer: A.**

Abnormal relaxation generally has normal LA pressure but an elevated LVEDP because of a combination of increased contribution of LV filling during atrial systole and possibly increased LV late diastolic stiffness by the same process that caused abnormal LV relaxation. Very high mean LA pressures result in pseudonormal or restrictive LV filling patterns.

Chapter 12

221. The following are potential complications of aortic valve endocarditis:
    A. Aortic root abscess
    B. Supra-annular mitral regurgitation
    C. Aneurysm of mitral–aortic intervalvular fibrosa
    D. Aneurysm of anterior mitral leaflet
    E. All of the above

222. The following statements are true about patent foramen ovale except:
    A. Pick-up rate is higher with saline contrast compared to color Doppler imaging
    B. Trans-esophageal echocardiogram (TEE) is more sensitive than transthoracic echocardiogram
    C. Yield is higher with leg injection compared to arm injection for saline contrast
    D. Present in about 40% of normal population

223. Saline contrast echocardiography in a patient with cirrhosis of the liver showed appearance of contrast in left atrium in five beats after its appearance in the right atrium. This is suggestive of:
    A. Normal physiology
    B. Hepatopulmonary syndrome
    C. Patent foramen ovale
    D. None of the above

224. Which type of aortic valve is least likely to be repairable for correction of severe aortic regurgitation?
    A. Failure of leaflet coaptation due to severely dilated ascending aorta with structurally normal leaflets
    B. Bicuspid aortic valve with prolapse of the conjoint cusp
    C. Aortic intramural hematoma with extension to the base of right coronary cusp causing it to prolapse
    D. Rheumatic aortic valve disease

225. TEE was performed intraoperatively following coronary artery bypass grafting (CABG) because of failure to wean from cardiopulmonary bypass. It showed akinetic inferior wall with 3 + mitral regurgitation originating at the medial commissure. These findings were not present preoperatively. The inferior wall looked excessively bright. Most likely problem in this patient is:
    A. Air embolism into right coronary artery (RCA)
    B. Thrombosis of RCA graft

   C. Excessively high blood pressure

   D. Excessive intravascular volume

   E. Poor myocardial preservation

226. The image is suggestive of:

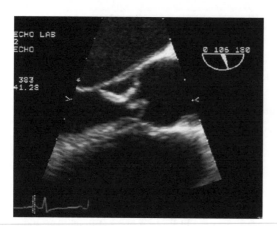

   A. Aortic dissection

   B. Aortic valve endocarditis

   C. Unicuspid aortic valve

   D. Hypertrophic cardiomyopathy

227. Continuous wave Doppler shown here could be a result of:

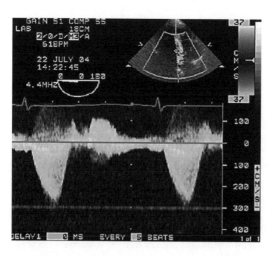

   A. Hypertrophic obstructive cardiomyopathy

   B. Severe mitral regurgitation

   C. Tricuspid regurgitation

   D. Ventricular septal defect

228. In this figure number "1" denotes:

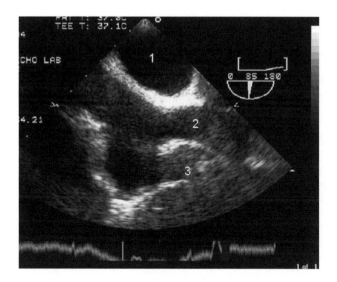

   A. Left atrium
   B. Right atrium
   C. Aorta
   D. Right pulmonary artery

229. In the figure number "2" is:

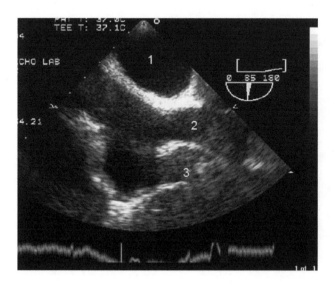

   A. Superior vena cava
   B. Inferior vena cava
   C. Pulmonary artery
   D. Aorta

230. In the figure number "3" denotes:

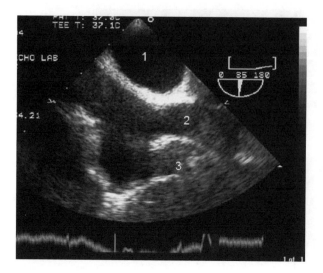

A. Left atrium

B. Right atrial appendage

C. Inferior vena cava

D. None of the above

231. This image shows:

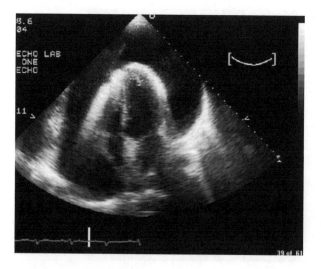

A. Large left pleural effusion

B. Large pericardial effusion with no evidence of tamponade

C. Large pericardial effusion with features of tamponade

D. Mirror image artifact

232. This mitral inflow pattern is consistent with:

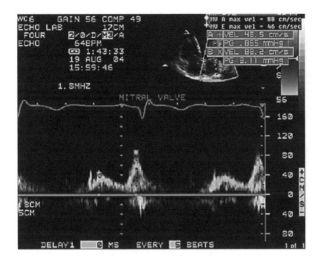

A. Abnormal left ventricular (LV) relaxation with elevated left atrial (LA) pressure
B. Abnormal LV relaxation with normal LA pressure
C. Pseudonormal filling
D. Restrictive LV filling

233. The part of the flow curve denoted by the arrow in this pulmonary vein flow is caused by:

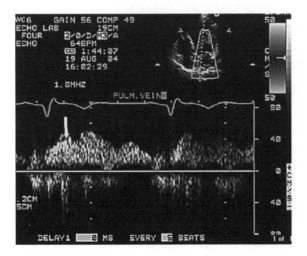

A. Left atrial relaxation
B. RV ejection
C. Mitral valve opening
D. Mitral annular descent

234. The patient shown here has:

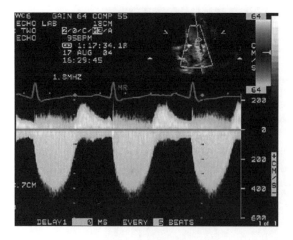

    A. Severe mitral regurgitation

    B. Severe mitral stenosis

    C. Severe aortic stenosis

    D. Mild mitral regurgitation

235. The mitral inflow pattern is consistent with:

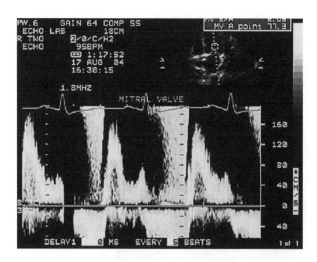

    A. Severe mitral regurgitation

    B. Severe mitral stenosis

    C. Prosthetic mitral valve

    D. Atrial fibrillation

236. In the image shown here the arrow denotes:

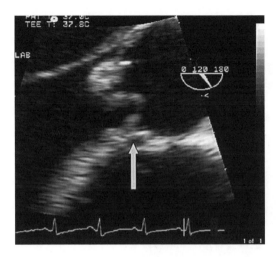

   A. Right coronary artery
   B. Coronary sinus
   C. Aortic ring abscess
   D. Prosthetic valve dehiscence

237. The aortic valve shown here is:

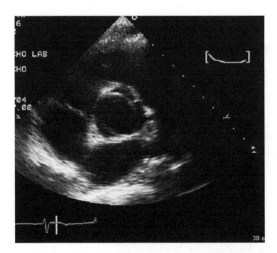

   A. Tricuspid
   B. Unicuspid
   C. Bicuspid with conjoint right and left cusp
   D. Bicuspid with conjoint left and noncoronary cusps

238. The TEE image shows:

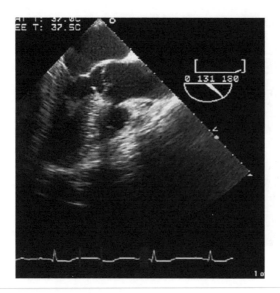

   A. Subaortic membrane
   B. Vegetation
   C. Artifact
   D. Aortic aneurysm

239. The Doppler signal is indicative of:

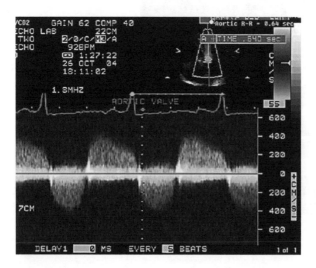

   A. Significant mixed aortic valve disease
   B. Significant mixed mitral valve disease
   C. Significant mixed tricuspid valve disease
   D. Hypertrophic obstructive cardiomyopathy

240. For the patient in the above question the LV end diastolic pressure is likely to be:
    A. Low
    B. Normal
    C. Elevated
    D. Cannot comment

Answers for chapter 12

221. **Answer: E.**

All of the above. In addition patients may get aorto-LV fistula, aorto-RV fistula, aorto-RA fistula, anterior mitral leaflet perforation, rupture of the mitral aortic intervalvular fibrosa, atrioventricular blocks, pyogenic pericarditis, etc.

222. **Answer: D.**

It is present in about 25% of the normal population.

223. **Answer: B.**

Due to the formation of pulmonary A–V fistulae (caused by "hepatic factor").

224. **Answer: D.**

For valve sparing surgery, leaflets should be structurally near normal.

225. **Answer: A.**

Akinetic wall signifies ischemia, and brightness indicates air embolism into RCA, the common artery to be affected because of its anterior origin from the aorta. Poor myocardial preservation would cause global hypokinesis. Mitral regurgitation (MR) in this patient is typically ischemic because of inferior wall motion abnormality.

226. **Answer: B.**

Large vegetations are seen on the aortic valve. Ascending aorta is normal sized with no visible flap. Unicuspid aortic valve can be diagnosed only in the short axis view showing only a single cusp and a single commissure.

227. **Answer: A.**

Late peaking systolic signal is indicative of dynamic LV outflow tract obstruction, which is most severe in end systole when the LV volume is minimal. The timing corresponds to LV ejection and begins following a period after the onset of the QRS signal. There is a gap between the end of the signal and onset of mitral inflow. The MR signal occupies not only the ejection period but also the isovolumic contraction and relaxation periods, is a longer signal and is continuous with the mitral inflow without any intervening gap. The tricuspid regurgitation (TR) signal is similar but tends to be broader with a lower velocity inflow. The cursor position, if visible, is also helpful to identify the origin of the signal. The ventricular septal defect signal is holosystolic but generally tends to have a presystolic component due to left atrial contraction.

228. **Answer: A.**

This TEE long axis view of the left atrium and right atrium is also popularly called a bicaval view; the left atrium is immediately anterior to the esophagus.

229. **Answer: A.**

In a vertical or near vertical plane, the right side is cephalad and the left side is caudal.

230. **Answer: B.**

Right atrial appendage.

231. **Answer: C.**
This figure shows pericardial effusion with features of tamponade (right atrial collapse).

232. **Answer: B.**
Abnormal LV relaxation pattern includes prolonged LV isovolumic relaxation time (>100 ms), E/A ratio < 1 and E-wave deceleration time > 250 ms.

233. **Answer: A.**
The arrow denotes the S1 wave, which is caused by left atrial relaxation. RV ejection and mitral annular descent generate the S2 wave, which follows the S1 wave. The mitral valve opening generates the D wave, which is synchronous with the mitral E wave.

234. **Answer: A.**
The timing of the signal starts with the QRS complex and the end, being continuous with the onset of mitral inflow, suggests MR. A density approaching that of mitral inflow suggests this to be severe. Other clues to severe MR could be a "V wave cut-off sign" and mitral inflow suggestive of high LA pressure.

235. **Answer: A.**
The presence of an A wave excludes atrial fibrillation, mitral stenosis and prosthetic mitral valve. The E-wave deceleration will be slow. The inflow pattern shown here indicates high left atrial pressure typified by E/A ratio > 2 and E-wave deceleration of <150 ms, and is consistent with severe MR.

236. **Answer: C.**
This patient has native aortic valve endocarditis with an anterior aortic ring abscess shown by the arrow. In patients with aortic valve endocarditis it is imperative to look for aortic root, ring or the mitral aortic intervalvular fibrosa. TEE is superior to transthoracic echocardiogram for this purpose.

237. **Answer: D.**
Bicuspid with conjoint left and noncoronary cusps.

238. **Answer: A.**
Note the membrane attached to the ventricular septum beneath the aortic valve. This is thin and uniformly membranous in appearance.

239. **Answer: A.**
The systolic signal does not begin with the onset of QRS, which is typical of MR or TR. Hence this is indicative of aortic stenosis (AS) with aortic regurgitation (AR). The AS signal is mid-peaking, which indicates a slow rise in aortic pressure. Note that the end of the AS signal is continuous with the AR signal, and vice versa. This indicates the origin of the signals at the same valve.

240. **Answer: C.**
Note the rapid deceleration of the AR signal and the late diastolic gradient between LV and aorta is only 16 mmHg when applying the simplified Bernoulli equation to the late diastolic AR velocity.

Chapter 13

241. This patient is likely to have:

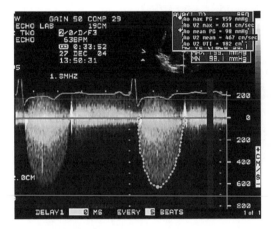

    A. Severe aortic stenosis (AS)

    B. Severe mitral regurgitation (MR)

    C. Severe pulmonary hypertension

    D. Mild AS

242. For the patient in question 241 the left ventricular outflow tract (LVOT) diameter was 2 cm and the LVOT velocity by pulse Doppler was 1 m/s. The aortic valve area by the continuity equation would be:

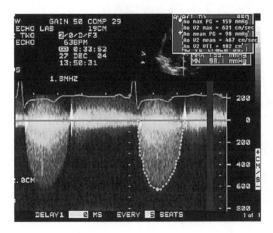

A. 0.2 cm^2

B. 0.3 cm^2

C. 0.5 cm^2

D. 0.8 cm^2

243. Image of the aortic arch shown here is indicative of:

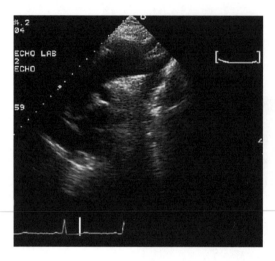

A. Aneurysm of the aortic arch

B. Aortic dissection

C. Severe coarctation of the aorta

D. Stented aortic coarctation

244. This is the continuous wave signal obtained from the pulmonary valve at the mid- to proximal esophageal location. This patient is likely to have:

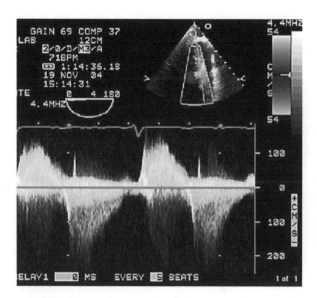

A. Wide open pulmonary regurgitation (PR)

B. Mild PR

C. Severe valvular pulmonary stenosis (PS)

D. Severe subvalvular PS

245. This patient has vegetation on:

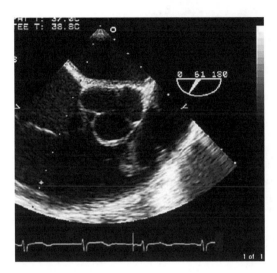

A. Aortic valve

B. Pulmonary valve

C. Tricuspid valve

D. Pacemaker lead

246. The appearance of the left atrial cavity is caused by:

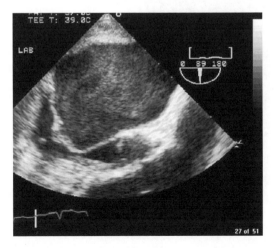

A. Stasis of blood

B. Mitral regurgitation

    C. Polycythemia

    D. Hyperdynamic circulation

247. The cause of the patient's mitral valve problem is:

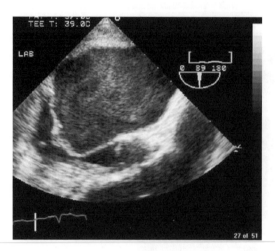

    A. Rheumatic heart disease

    B. Degenerative valve disease

    C. Fen Phen valvulopathy

    D. Ischemic heart disease

248. The arrow in this image points to:

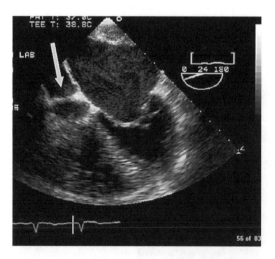

    A. Right atrium (RA)

    B. Coronary sinus

   C. Left atrium (LA)

   D. Right ventricle (RV)

249. The arrow in this image points to:

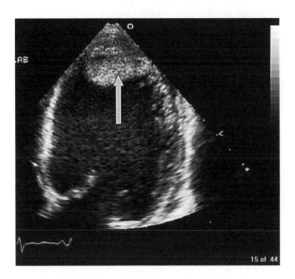

   A. Left ventricular (LV) apical thrombus

   B. RV thrombus

   C. Rib artifact

   D. LA thrombus

250. This patient is likely to have:

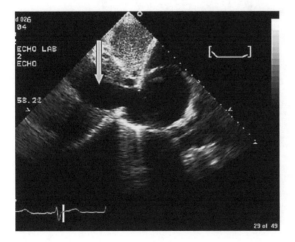

   A. High RA pressure

   B. Pericardial effusion

   C. Aortic dissection

   D. Dilated azygos vein

251. The pulmonary vein flow shown here is indicative of:

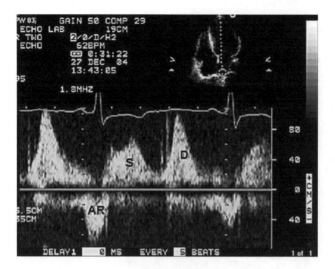

A. Elevated LA pressure with normal end diastolic pressure (EDP)

B. Elevated LA pressure with elevated EDP

C. Abnormal LV relaxation with normal EDP

D. Elevated LVEDP with normal LA pressure

252. The mitral flow pattern shown here is suggestive of:

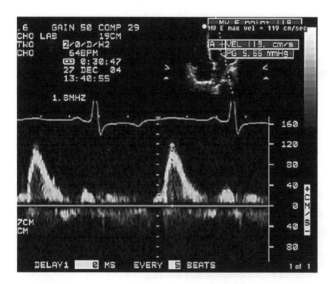

A. Normal LA pressure

B. High LA pressure

C. Atrial mechanical failure

D. Abnormal LV relaxation with normal LA pressure

253. This patient has:

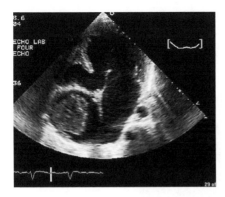

A. Mitral atresia

B. Tricuspid atresia

C. Transposition of great vessels with atrial baffle

D. Epstein's anomaly

254. The structure denoted by the arrow is likely to be:

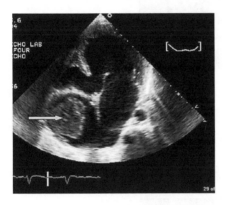

A. Artifact

B. Right atrial thrombus

C. Myxoma

D. Fibroelastoma

255. This patient in likely to have:

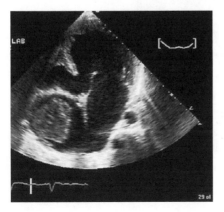

A. Normal pulmonary artery (PA) flow

B. Pulmonary hypertension approaching systemic pressure

C. Nonsignificant amount of flow from RV to PA

D. None of the above

256. This patient has:

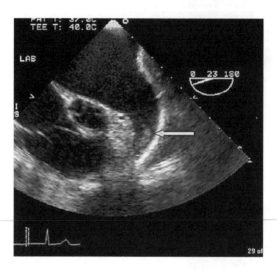

A. Normal LA appendage

B. Clot in the LA appendage

C. Tumor in the LA appendage

D. None of the above

257. This patient has:

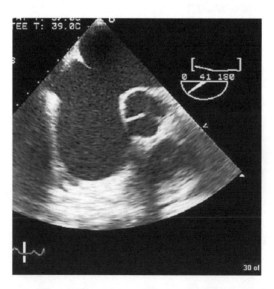

A. Prominent Eustachian valve

B. Ostium secundum atrial septal defect (ASD)

C. Ostium primum ASD

D. Sinus venosus ASD

258. What type of flow was recorded from the mid-esophageal position?

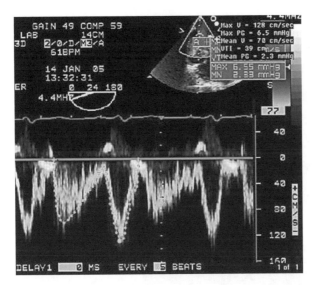

A. Mitral flow

B. Pulmonary vein flow

C. Superior vena cava flow

D. Flow across ASD

259. This patient has a secundum ASD with dimensions of the defect 3 × 2 cm, time velocity integral (TVI) of flow across the defect is 39 cm and the heart rate is 70/s. The approximate shunt flow across the ASD is:

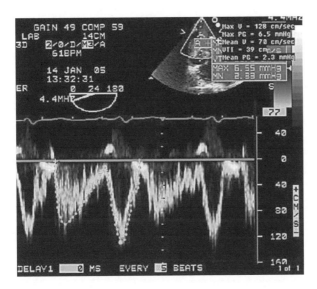

A. 12.8 L/min

B. 3 L/min

C. 7 L/min

D. Cannot be calculated

260. This patient has:

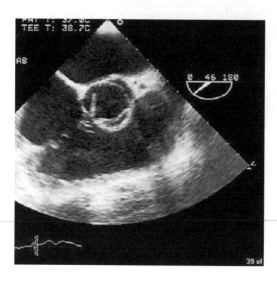

A. Aortic stenosis

B. Normal opening trileaflet aortic valve

C. Bicuspid aortic valve that opens well

D. Unicommissural aortic valve

Answers for chapter 13

241. **Answer: A.**

This is an AS signal. Please pay attention to the onset of the signal. Typically a peak gradient > 80 mmHg and a mean gradient of 40 mmHg are indicative of severe AS, though they are flow dependent. Valve area is a better indicator of severity of AS.

242. **Answer: C.**

By the continuity equation $A_1V_1 = A_2V_2$. Hence the aortic valve area $(A_2 = A_1V_1/V_2) = 3.14 \times 1 \times 1 \times 1/6 = 0.5\,\text{cm}^2$ approximately.

243. **Answer: D.**

Note the increased density of the aortic wall in the area of coarctation. This represents the stent.

244. **Answer: A.**

Note the rapid deceleration of the PR signal with rapid equilibration of late diastolic PA and RV pressures. The increased systolic flow velocity is due to increased flow secondary to wide open PR.

245. **Answer: B.**

Pulmonary valve.

246. **Answer: A.**

This is a spontaneous echo contrast, indicating low velocity of flow, predisposes to thrombus formation and is a marker of embolic risk. Intensity of spontaneous echo contrast is affected by the velocity of blood flow and is exaggerated with higher gain settings and a higher transducer frequency.

247. **Answer: A.**

Patient has classic rheumatic mitral stenosis. The anterior leaflet is thin with a hockey-stick appearance in diastole, which occurs due to commissural fusion. In degenerative MS there is severe annular calcification, which extends into the leaflets causing stenosis. In fen Phen valvulopathy leaflets are thick and fibrosed and may result in both MS and MR. Ischemic involvement of the LV without papillary muscle rupture causes restriction of closure and functional MR and not mitral stenosis.

248. **Answer: A.**

Right atrium.

249. **Answer: A.**

The position of the septal leaflet of the tricuspid valve confirms the chamber in question to be the left ventricle.

250. **Answer: A.**

The inferior vena cava as confirmed by its connection to the right atrium is dilated and is about 2.5 cm in diameter This indicates high RA pressure, especially if associated with reduced collapse with inspiration. Patients on ventilators may have a dilated inferior vena cava (IVC) without high RA pressure. Young patients might have a dilated IVC with collapse on inspiration, which is normal.

251. **Answer: B.**

The rapid D-wave deceleration with time < 170 ms indicates high LA pressure. In addition, the S wave is smaller than the D wave. The atrial regurgitation (AR) wave duration is about 220 ms. The normal duration is about 80–100 ms. This is due to increased duration of atrial systole having to pump against elevated LVEDP. Pulmonary vein AR duration greater than mitral A-wave duration is indicative of high LVEDP.

252. **Answer: B.**

This inflow pattern shows high E/A ratio. The deceleration time is also short, suggestive of high LA pressure. In pure atrial mechanical failure the E wave is normal, with diminished mitral A-wave amplitude.

253. **Answer: B.**

The atretic tricuspid valve is shown. There was no ASD and outflow from RA was through right atrium to pulmonary artery shunt. Patient also had superior vena caval-right pulmonary artery shunt. Both were patent.

254. **Answer: B.**

Right atrial thrombus in this patient with tricuspid atresia. Because of atriopulmonary shunt, there is right atrial stasis.

255. **Answer: C.**

There is tricuspid atresia and pulmonary flow is occurring through cavopulmonary or atriopulmonary shunt in the absence of an ASD. This would need low pulmonary vascular resistance and low PA pressure. This patient has a nonrestrictive ventricular septal defect and hence RV systolic pressure would be the same as LV systolic pressure and to maintain low PA pressure the RV outflow should be minimal or nonexistent. In this patient this was accomplished surgically with banding of the pulmonary artery.

256. **Answer: B.**

This patient has a clot in the LA appendage. This is best visualized with a transesophageal echocardiogram from an upper esophageal location. The appendage may be multilobed and it is important to examine it in multiple tomographic planes.

257. **Answer: B.**

Ostium secundum ASD. Primum ASD would be in the lower part of the septum and may involve anterior mitral leaflet and A–V conduction. Sinus venosus ASD is in the upper septum near the superior vena cava and may also be associated with anomalous drainage of the right upper pulmonary vein. There is also a rare type of sinus venosus ASD in the vicinity of the IVC. In unroofed coronary sinus, the shunt is from LA to RA through a posterior defect into the coronary sinus such that flow goes through the coronary sinus into the RA.

258. **Answer: D.**

This biphasic flow with a systolic-early diastolic component and LA contraction is typical of ASD flow. Pulmonary vein flow and superior vena cava flow would be triphasic, with distinct systolic and diastolic flows with reversal and atrial contraction. Mitral flow has only diastolic components with early and late diastolic components.

259. **Answer: A.**

The shunt flow per beat can be calculated as the product of the TVI of the shunt flow and the anatomic area of the defect. This would be $39 \times 3.14 \times 1.5 \times 1$ cc/beat (183 cc). This multiplied by the heart rate gives the shunt flow per minute.

260. **Answer: B.**

Normal opening of the trileaflet aortic valve.

Chapter 14

Questions

261. The arrow here points to:

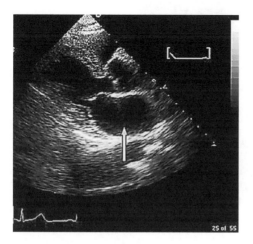

A. Left atrium

B. Right pulmonary artery

C. Posterior pericardial effusion

D. Left pleural effusion

262. The structure denoted by the arrow is:

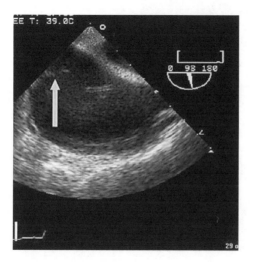

A. Vegetation

B. Eustachian valve

C. Edge of atrial septal defect (ASD)

D. Tricuspid valve

263. The structure shown by the arrow is:

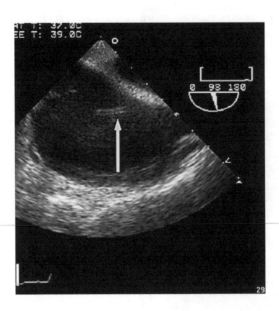

A. Artifact

B. Catheter in right atrium

C. Thrombus

D. Loose suture material

264. The patient may have all of the following except:

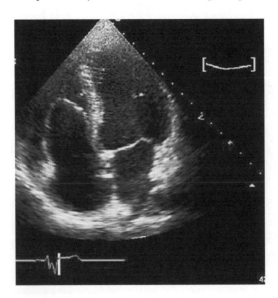

A. Atrial septal defect

B. Wolf–Parkinson–White syndrome

C. Tricuspid regurgitation

D. Bicuspid aortic valve

265. The mitral valve abnormality seen here is:

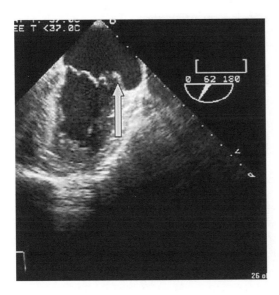

A. Perforation, prolapse of P1 scallop of posterior leaflet

B. Abnormal P3 scallop

C. Prolapsing P2 scallop

D. Anterior leaflet prolapse

266. The structure denoted here is:

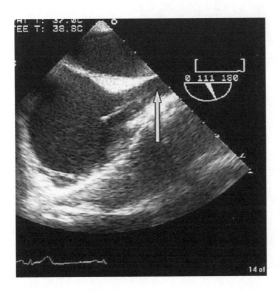

A. Superior vena cava

B. Inferior vena cava

C. Right upper pulmonary vein

D. Main pulmonary artery

267. The numbers 1, 2 and 3 denote the following cusps of the aortic valve:

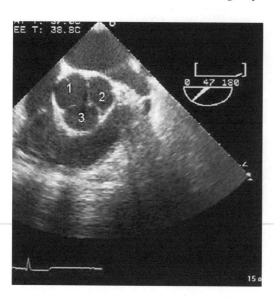

A. Nonleft right coronary

B. Left, right, noncoronary

C. Right, left, noncoronary

D. Noncoronary, right, left

268. Structure no. 4 denotes:

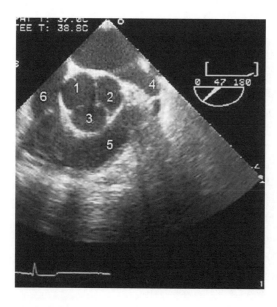

A. Left atrial appendage
B. Right atrial appendage
C. Left upper pulmonary vein
D. Left lower pulmonary vein

269. The structure shown by the arrow is:

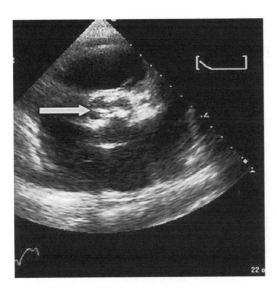

A. Calcified native aortic valve
B. Stented bioprosthetic aortic valve
C. St. Jude bileaflet mechanical aortic valve
D. Supravalvular aortic stenosis as part of William's syndrome

270. The M-mode echocardiogram is suggestive of:

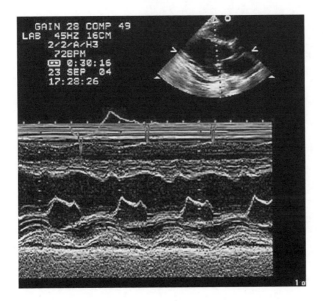

A. Normal mitral valve motion

B. Mitral stenosis

C. Severe aortic regurgitation

D. High left atrial pressure

271. The image shown here is suggestive of:

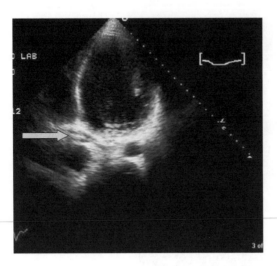

A. Mitral annuloplasty

B. Catheter in the coronary artery

C. Biventricular pacemaker

D. An artifact

272. The structure denoted by the arrow is:

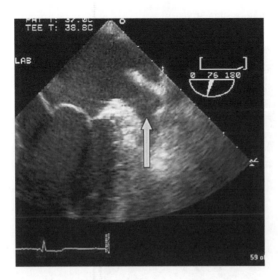

A. Left atrial appendage

B. Left lower pulmonary vein

C. Left upper pulmonary vein

D. Right lower pulmonary vein

273. The patient shown here has:

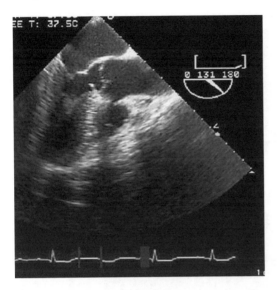

A. Valvular aortic stenosis

B. Subvalvular aortic stenosis

C. Endocarditis

D. Hypertrophic obstructive cardiomyopathy

274. The arrow is indicative of:

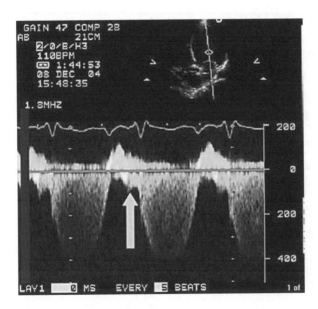

A. Diastolic mitral regurgitation

B. An artifact

    C. Pulmonary vein D wave picked up by the continuous wave cursor

    D. Mitral annular motion superimposed on the mitral flow

275. This patient is likely to have:

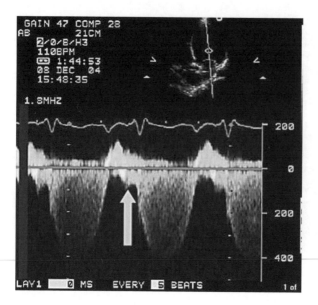

    A. Systolic heart failure

    B. Flail mitral valve with good left ventricular function

    C. Isolated severe acute aortic regurgitation

    D. None of the above

276. This patient is likely to have:

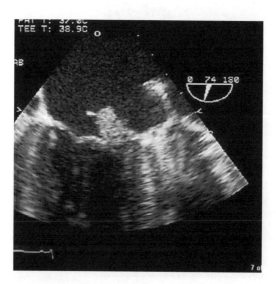

    A. Papillary muscle rupture

    B. Mitral valve endocarditis

C. Fibroelastoma

D. Libman–Sacks endocarditis

277. The need for surgical intervention in this patient is:

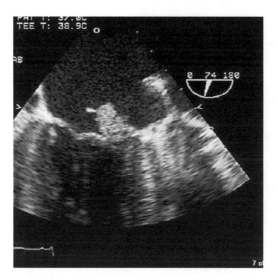

A. Low

B. Intermediate

C. High

D. This is a nonsurgical condition

278. The structure denoted by the arrow is:

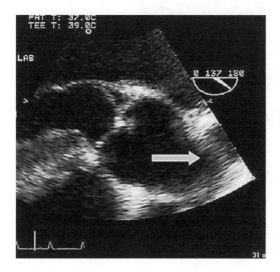

A. Ascending aorta

B. Main pulmonary artery

C. Right atrium

D. Right ventricular outflow tract

279. The structure indicated by the arrow is:

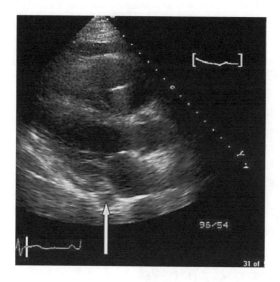

    A. Descending thoracic aorta
    B. Coronary sinus
    C. Inferior vena cava
    D. Circumflex coronary artery

280. The arrow indicates:

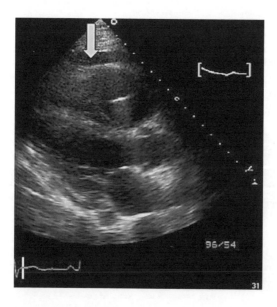

    A. Pleural effusion
    B. Pericardial effusion
    C. Pericardial pad of fat
    D. Artifact

Answers for chapter 14

261. **Answer: A.**

Left atrium

262. **Answer: B.**

The structure is the Eustachian valve. In the vertical plane the inferior vena cava (IVC) is caudal and gets displayed to the left side of the monitor.

263. **Answer: B.**

This structure has a double wall with a central lumen, which is suggestive of a catheter. In addition the structure is linear. Suture material will not have a lumen and thrombus is not uniform in diameter and has no central lucency.

264. **Answer: D.**

This patient has Epstein's anomaly. Note the downward displacement of the septal leaflet of the tricuspid valve compared to the mitral leaflet attachment. A displacement of >8 mm/M2 is suggestive of Epstein's. The septal leaflet may be large, sail-like and adherent to the ventricular septum. This is frequently associated with ASD, right-sided accessory pathway and tricuspid regurgitation, but not bicuspid aortic valve.

265. **Answer: A.**

In this intercommissural view obtained at about 70°, the area denoted by the arrow is the lateral or P1 scallop of the posterior mitral leaflet. P3 is at the medial commissure. Generally the A2 scallop, i.e. middle scallop of the anterior leaflet, is seen in the middle. However, if the probe is rotated counterclockwise to the left the P2 scallop may be seen in this location.

266. **Answer: A.**

This is a long axis image through the superior vena cana (SVC) and the right atrium. Advancing the probe further down the esophagus will show the bicaval view. Left atrium is seen closer to the transducer, separated by the atrial septum from the right atrium. Rightward or clockwise rotation will display the right upper pulmonary vein, and leftward or counterclockwise rotation will show the ascending aorta.

267. **Answer: A.**

Note that the probe is in the esophagus and the anterior is away from the transducer, contrary to the short axis view of the aortic valve by transthoracic echocardiogram.

268. **Answer: A.**

This structure is the left atrial appendage. Structure no. 5 is the right ventricular outflow tract and structure no. 6 is the right atrium.

269. **Answer: A.**

This is a calcified native aortic valve. The native leaflets are seen. There are no struts of a bioprosthetic valve visible. A mechanical valve produces intense shadowing with poor visualization of the disc unless an end-on view is obtained.

270. **Answer: A.**

This M mode is suggestive of normal mitral valve motion. There is normal mitral valve opening with greater early diastolic opening compared to opening associated with left atrial contraction. Valvular mitral stenosis would cause mitral leaflet thickening, reduced opening and reduced ejection fraction (EF) slope and paradoxical anterior motion of the posterior leaflet during diastole because of commissural fusion. Severe aortic regurgitation (AR) may cause fluttering of the anterior mitral leaflet and premature closure of the anterior mitral leaflet as the mitral valve opening is flow dependent. Features of high left atrial pressure will include predominant early opening, rapid EF slope and a smaller opening with atrial contraction mirroring the transmitral inflow pattern.

271. **Answer: C.**

The arrow here depicts a lead in the coronary sinus and is consistent with a biventricular pacemaker.

272. **Answer: A.**

The structure denoted by the arrow is the left atrial appendage. This is separated from the left upper pulmonary vein, which is to the posterior with a ridge popularly known as the "coumadin ridge" because of the potential to be misinterpreted as a thrombus. Because this ridge is echoreflective, sometimes one can see thrombus-like artifacts in the appendage as mirror image artifacts. Though the appendage is clearly visualized here, this view alone is not sufficient to rule out a thrombus. Multiple tomographic views have to be obtained through the appendage in its entirety as the appendage may have multiple lobes.

273. **Answer: B.**

The structure attached to the septum below the aortic valve is a classic subaortic membrane. Occasionally vegetations can be seen here due to seeding from the aortic valve. This is a diastolic frame and hence aortic valve opening cannot be evaluated.

274. **Answer: A.**

This is diastolic mitral regurgitation (MR), which in this patient is probably due to high left venticular end diastolic pressure (LVEDP) or coexistent severe AR. Other causes of diastolic MR include prolonged PR interval, prolonged A–V delay or A–V dissociation. The velocity of this signal is about 1.2 m/s, which is high for tissue velocity. Pulmonary vein D wave would be in the opposite direction, i.e. in the direction of the mitral E wave.

275. **Answer: A.**

The profile of MR is indicative of severe LV systolic dysfunction in view of prolonged duration of the MR signal and severely reduced dp/dt in the presence of normal QRS duration. In this example the time taken for the MR velocity to rise from 1m/s to 3 m/s is 60 ms, which translates into an LV positive dp/dt of 530 mmHg/s (32/0.06). Also note that the diastolic filling period is short and the diastolic MR in this patient is likely from high LVEDP, as the PR interval is not unduly prolonged.

276. **Answer: B.**

There is a large mass attached to the P1 scallop of the mitral valve with a soft tissue characteristic less echo dense than the mitral leaflets and a secondary thin mass attached to this. The attachment of this lesion is to the atrial side of the mitral leaflet. This is highly consistent with vegetation. Nonbacterial vegetation of Libman-Sacks endocarditis is a complication of systemic lupus erythematosus and is generally smaller, multiple and verrucous. Fibroelastomas are more echodense, nodular, generally pedunculated and mobile, usually attached to the ventricular side of the mitral valve.

277. **Answer: C.**

The vegetation is very large, measuring about 1.5×1 cm, and has a high embolic potential in view of its mobility, large size and mobile elements attached to its tip. It also has a high potential for lack of bacterial clearance with antibiotics alone because of the size. In addition this patient has severe mitral regurgitation. In general the indications for surgery include: lack of response to medical therapy, valvular disruption, recurrent embolization, abscess formation, fungal vegetations. Size greater than 1 cm is a relative indication for surgery because of the potential for complications.

278. **Answer: A.**

Ascending aorta.

279. **Answer: B.**

This structure is in the posterior A–V groove, is intrapericardial and is markedly dilated. Dilatation can occur as a result of either increased flow or increased pressure. Causes include persistent left SVC, right heart failure, coronary fistula and unroofed coronary sinus. Descending thoracic aorta is extrapericardial. Hence if there is a pericardial effusion, it would be anterior to the aorta and pleural effusion would be posterior to the aorta. This degree of aneurysm of circumflex artery is unusual. The IVC does not course this area.

280. **Answer: B.**

This echolucent space is clearly between two layers of the pericardium. The space is totally echolucent, which indicates fluid rather than fat tissue.

Chapter 15

281. This image shows a vegetation on the:

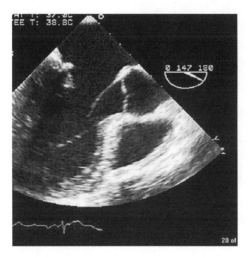

A. Aortic valve
B. P2 scallop of mitral valve
C. P1 scallop of mitral valve
D. A2 scallop of mitral valve

282. The hemodynamics in this patient potentially could be improved by:

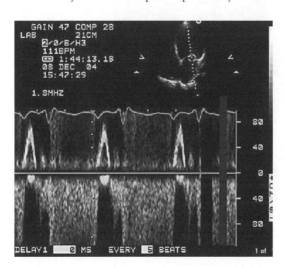

    A. Shortening the PR interval

    B. Afterload reduction

    C. Positive inotropes

    D. All of the above

283. The trans-esophageal echocardiogram (TEE) image shown here is indicative of:

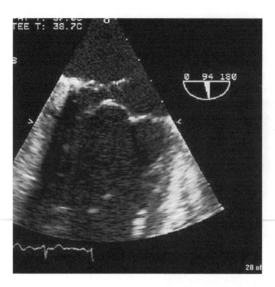

    A. Flail posterior leaflet P3 segment

    B. Flail posterior leaflet P1 segment

    C. Flail anterior leaflet

    D. Large mitral valve vegetation

284. The pulse wave Doppler in the right upper pulmonary vein is indicative of:

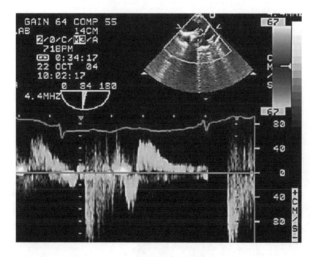

    A. Abnormal left ventricular (LV) relaxation

    B. High left atrial (LA) pressure

C. Mitral stenosis

D. Severe mitral regurgitation (MR)

285. This apical four-chamber view shows:

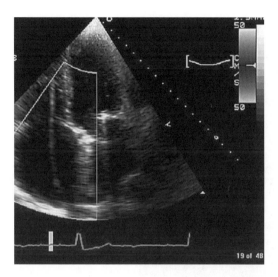

A. A pacemaker lead in the right ventricle (RV)

B. A pacemaker lead in the coronary sinus

C. Epicardial RV lead

D. Artifact in the RV

286. The mitral valve opening pattern in this patient is suggestive of:

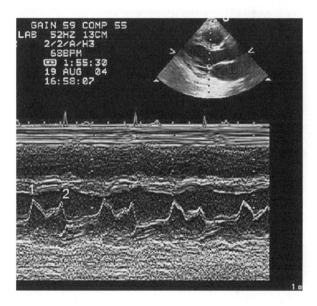

A. Mitral stenosis

B. High left ventricular end diastolic pressure (LVEDP)

    C. Atrial fibrillation

    D. Normal pattern

287. The part of the anatomy and measurement indicated by the line is:

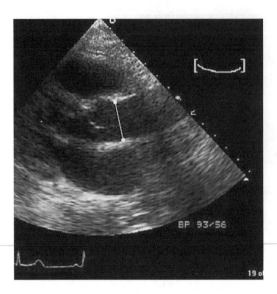

    A. The sino-tubular junction

    B. Sinus diameter

    C. Sinus height

    D. Aortic annular diameter

288. The blood supply to the ventricular septum shown here is:

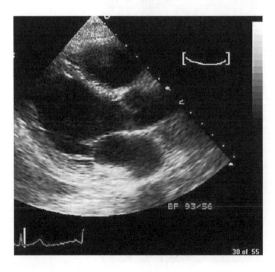

    A. Left anterior descending (LAD)

    B. Patent ductus arteriosus

C. Both

D. Neither

289. The structure indicated by the arrow in the ascending aorta is likely to be:

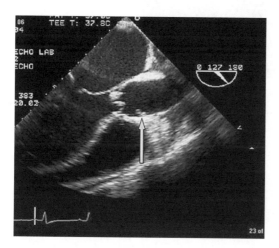

A. Vegetative aortitis

B. Flap of aortic dissection

C. Intraaortic atherosclerotic debris

D. Supravalvular aortic stenosis

290. The structure indicated by the arrow is likely to be:

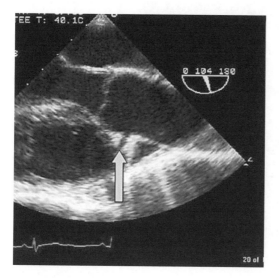

A. Aortic dissection

B. Aortic transaction

C. Right coronary artery

D. Left coronary artery

291. The arrow in this short axis view transthoracic echocardiogram (TTE) image at the level of the ascending aorta is:

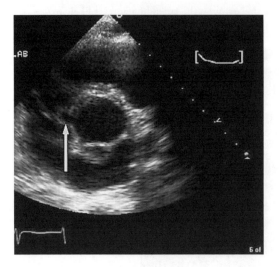

A. Artifact

B. Tissue plane and aorta and RV outflow tract

C. Aortic dissection

D. Right coronary artery

292. The structure shown by the arrow is:

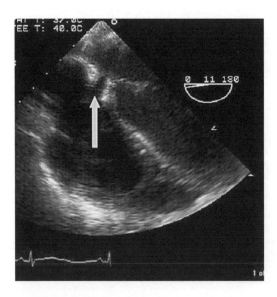

A. Coronary sinus

B. Atrial septal defect (ASD)

C. Superior vena cava

D. Inferior vena cava

293. The valve indicated by the arrow is:

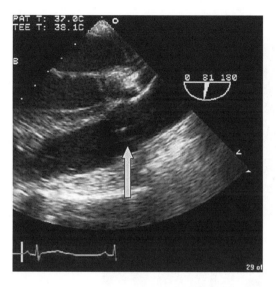

    A. Pulmonary valve

    B. Aortic valve

    C. Tricuspid valve

    D. Mirror image artifact of the aortic valve

294. This view is obtained from the upper esophagus. The structure indicated by the arrow is:

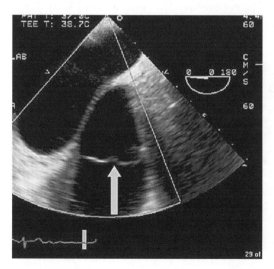

    A. Aortic valve

    B. Pulmonary valve

    C. Tricuspid valve

    D. Artifact

295. The pulmonary regurgitation signal shown here is indicative of (assuming right atrial pressure of 15 mmHg):

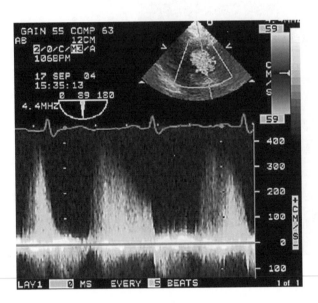

   A. Normal pulmonary artery (PA) pressure
   B. Mild pulmonary hypertension
   C. Moderate pulmonary hypertension
   D. None of the above

296. This subcostal view shows part of the liver. This patient has a history of episodes of flushing and diarrhea. The likely diagnosis is:

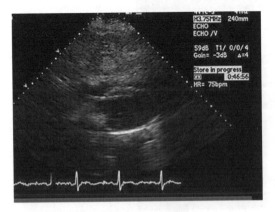

   A. Amebic liver abscess
   B. Right atrial myxoma
   C. Carcinoid syndrome
   D. Renal cell carcinoma

297. This 86-year-old patient has intractable heart failure and chronic atrial fibrillation. The finding on the still image is suggestive of:

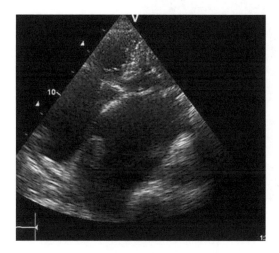

    A. Left atrial thrombus
    B. Lipomatous atrial septum
    C. ASD closure device
    D. Side lobe artifact

298. In question 297 the left ventricular size and ejection fraction were normal. The patient is likely to have:

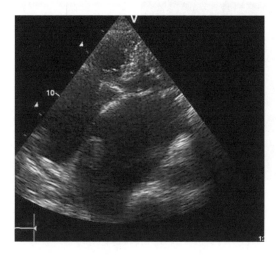

    A. Restrictive cardiomyopathy
    B. Congestive cardiomyopathy
    C. Hypertrophic cardiomyopathy
    D. None of the above

299. The short axis image of this patient shows:

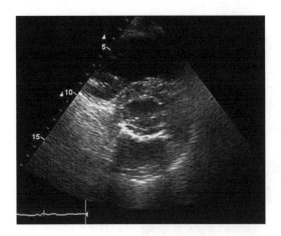

    A. Posterior pericardial effusion

    B. Massive mitral annular calcification

    C. Calcified aortic valves

    D. None of the above

300. The appearance of the interatrial septum is indicative of:

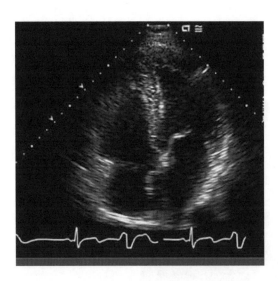

    A. Left atrial myxoma

    B. Aneurysmal atrial septum

    C. ASD

    D. None of the above

Answers for chapter 15

281. **Answer: B.**

This is a long axis cut through the mitral valve, which courses through the middle of both the anterior and posterior leaflets and hence would show A2 and P2 scallops, respectively. Pushing the probe down will cut through A3 and P3 scallops and pulling the probe up will cut through A1 and P1 scallops.

282. **Answer: D.**

Note that this patient has a markedly dilated LV and very short diastole despite a heart rate of about 70/min, very premature atrial contraction with no passive transmitral flow, with diastolic MR and prolonged systole as indicated by the systolic MR signal. All of these indicate poor systolic performance and AV dysynchrony. Hence the hemodynamics is likely to improve with the therapies listed above. The QRS duration in the monitored ECG is 100 ms. However 12-lead ECG has to be examined for QRS duration. If QRS duration is prolonged, or mechanical asynchrony is demonstrated by echocardiography, then the patient may also benefit from biventricular pacing.

283. **Answer: A.**

This patient has a flail P3 scallop of the posterior mitral leaflet. In this near intercommissural view, with slight rightward rotation, the scallops from right to left include A1, A2 and P3. At about a 70–80° angle the scallops seen would be P1, A2 and P3. At around 120–130° the scallops seen would be A2 and P2.

284. **Answer: D.**

This is severe MR. Note the holosystolic flow reversal in the pulmonary vein.

285. **Answer: A.**

This is an RV endocardial lead. The coronary sinus (CS) is not visualized here. The CS leads tend to be thinner. CS can be imaged with a posterior tilt from this plane. The ICD leads are much thicker than the pacer leads.

286. **Answer: D.**

This is an M-mode through the mitral valve showing a normal pattern with E(1) and A(2) waves on the image of normal amplitude and movement of the posterior leaflet, which is a mirror image in the opposite direction. In atrial fibrillation the A wave disappears. High LVEDP is classically characterized by a "B" hump, which is a positive deflection on the downslope of the A wave. Features of mitral stenosis include mitral leaflet thickening, reduced opening, flatter, ejection fraction slope and paradoxical anterior motion of the posterior leaflet during diastole due to leaflet fusion.

287. **Answer: A.**

This is the sino-tubular junction (STJ), which is the junction between the sinus and the tubular portions of ascending aorta. This diameter is usually less than the annulus diameter. The sinus height is the distance between the annulus and the ST junction and is increased in conditions that, cause aneurysmal dilatation of the sinus portion of the aorta. Excessive dilatation of the STJ may cause restriction in the closure of the aortic valve and may result in aortic regurgitation in the absence of leaflet pathology and in the presence of normal annulus size. This can be corrected by restoration of the aortic root anatomy with root replacement.

288. **Answer: A.**

The entire ventricular septum seen here is anterior, supplied by the LAD artery. The first septal perforator of the LAD artery supplies the very proximal septum.

289. **Answer: A.**

This thin filamentous mass in association with aortic valve vegetation was vegetation on the aortic wall seeding the right side of the aortic wall as a jet lesion. There is no false lumen or intramural hematoma to support the diagnosis of a flap. The remainder of the aorta is normal without any atherosclerotic changes, however a small atheromatous mass is still a possibility.

290. **Answer: C.**

This is anterior and the artery is coming out of the right sinus of valsalva on this TEE. Dissection will be characterized by a thin mobile flap and a false lumen. In transection, there would be a thicker, localized flap protruding into the aortic lumen associated with disruption of media and adventitia.

291. **Answer: D.**

Note the tubular nature of the structure and its continuity with the aortic lumen. Right coronary artery arises anteriorly from this location and the origin of the left coronary artery would be in the 4 o'clock position (not shown here).

292. **Answer: A.**

This low esophageal view at the gastro–esophageal junction with the transverse plane in the A–V groove posteriorly demonstrates the coronary sinus draining into the right atrium. A long axis cut through the vena cavae is generally seen in the vertical bicaval view in the 80–120° angle.

293. **Answer: A.**

Note that this is anterior and connects to the PA. Also seen is part of the aortic valve posterior to this structure.

294. **Answer: B.**

The structure indicated by the arrow is the pulmonary valve. The structure closer to the transducer is the aortic arch in transverse plane. Part of the main PA is seen closer to the transducer.

295. **Answer: C.**

The end diastolic velocity is 2.1 m/s, which translates into an end diastolic gradient of 17 mmHg between the PA and the RV. Assuming the RVEDP to be the same as the mean RA pressure of 15 mmHg, the computed PA end diastolic pressure would be 32 mmHg. This is consistent with moderate to severe pulmonary hypertension. Also note that the PR signal is rapidly decelerating, indicating either severe PR or rapidly increasing RVEDP.

296. **Answer: C.**

The image shows abnormal liver with a multiple echogenic and echoluscent area consistent with metastatic tumor. This combined with the clinical presentation is indicative of carcinoid syndrome. Valves most commonly affected include the tricuspid and pulmonary valves. Renal cell carcinoma extends to the heart through the inferior vena cava. Right atrial myxoma usually is attached to the atrial septum or the atrial free wall.

297. **Answer: A.**

This is a left atrial thrombus. A large mass is visualized attached to the atrial septum in the fossa ovalis area. In the given clinical context this is likely to be a thrombus. Differential diagnosis includes left atrial myxoma. Lipomatous atrial septum spares the fossa ovalis but causes thickening of the rest of the septum due to fat deposition. An ASD closure device like the Amplatzer device has a characteristic internal architecture made up of mesh and wires.

298. **Answer: A.**

Severe biatrial enlargement with a normal sized ventricle associated with high filling pressures is diagnostic of restrictive cardiomyopathy. This patient has aneurysmal biatrial enlargement. This patient also had low voltage electrocardiographic complexes, which is suggestive of cardiac amyloidosis.

299. **Answer: B.**

The posterior annulus is massively calcified. The echolucent area posterior to this is due to shadowing because of lack of penetration through this massively calcified structure.

300. **Answer: B.**

The fossa ovalis is bowing towards the right atrium. This back and forth movement of the fossa is better visualized during dynamic imaging. This is associated with patent foramen ovale and increased risk of stroke and possibly migraine. The image does not show any mass or atrial septal defect, though a tangential cut through the aneurysmal septum may mimic a mass in certain views during dynamic imaging.

Chapter 16

Questions

301. The parasternal long axis image of the mitral valve apparatus shows:

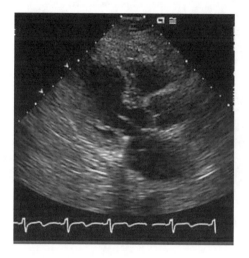

    A. Mitral annular calcification

    B. Rheumatic mitral stenosis

    C. Systolic anterior motion

    D. Annuloplasty ring

302. The continuous wave signal shown here is indicative of:

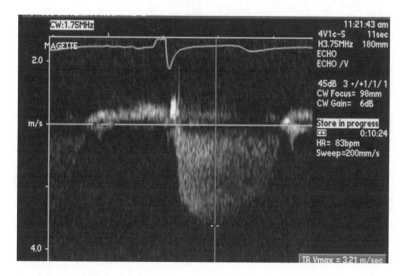

A. Moderate aortic stenosis

B. Moderate pulmonary hypertension

C. Acute severe mitral regurgitation due to papillary muscle rupture

D. None of the above

303. Assuming a right atrial (RA) pressure of 10 mmHg, the pulmonary regurgitation signal shown here is indicative of:

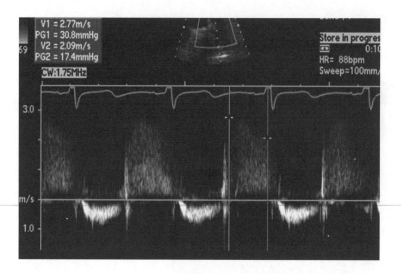

A. Normal pulmonary artery (PA) pressure

B. Moderate elevation of PA pressure

C. Systemic level of PA pressure

D. None of the above

304. The abnormalities shown in this image include:

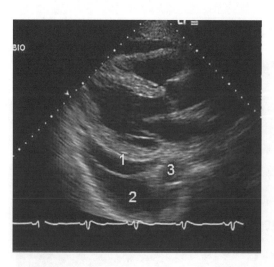

A. Pericardial effusion

B. Left pleural effusion

C. Left pleural effusion and pericardial effusion

D. Abnormally thick pericardium

305. The pattern of aortic valve opening in this patient is likely to be due to:

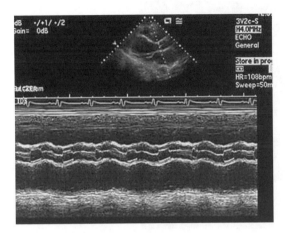

A. Hypertrophic obstructive cardiomyopathy (HOCM)

B. Pulsus alternans

C. Intra-aortic balloon pump (IABP) with 1:3 support

D. Left ventricular assist device (LVAD) with 1:3 support

306. This is an apical four-chamber view of the left ventricle (LV). The structure indicated by the arrow in the LV apex is likely to be:

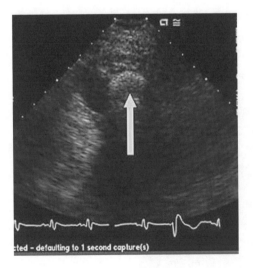

A. LV thrombus

B. Rib artifact

C. Cannula of LVAD

D. False tendon in the LV apex

307. The structure indicated by the arrow is:

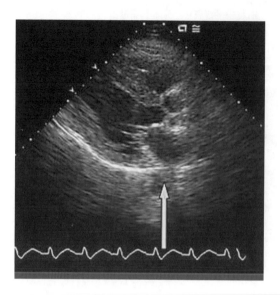

A. Descending thoracic aorta
B. Coronary sinus
C. Left lower pulmonary vein
D. Left PA

308. The transthoracic image shown here is indicative of:

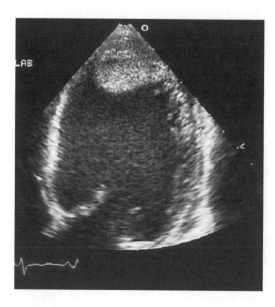

A. LV apical thrombus
B. Moderator band

   C. Rib artifact

   D. Ventricular non-compaction

309. The patient shown here is likely to have:

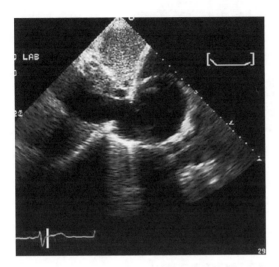

   A. Heart failure

   B. Intravascular volume depletion with hypotension

   C. Right atrial tumor

   D. None of the above

310. The continuous wave Doppler signal shown here is suggestive of:

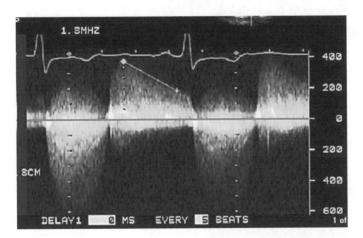

   A. Mixed mitral valve disease with significant mitral stenosis (MS) and mitral regurgitation (MR)

   B. Mixed aortic valve disease with significant aortic stenosis (AS) and atrial regurgitation (AR)

   C. Combination of AR and MR

   D. Ventricular septal defect (VSD) with bidirectional flow

311. This patient is likely to have (BP 130/65 mmHg):

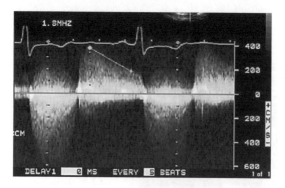

   A. High left ventricular end diastolic pressure (LVEDP)
   B. Diastolic MR
   C. Premature mitral valve closure
   D. All of the above

312. The following statements are true of the Doppler signal shown here:

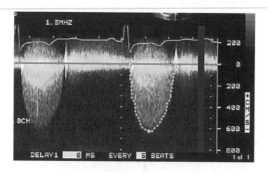

   A. The patient may have severe valvular aortic stenosis
   B. The patient may have severe systolic anterior motion (SAM)
   C. Patient may have severe MR
   D. None of the above

313. The pulmonary vein flow pattern is indicative of:

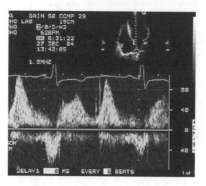

A. Volume depletion

B. Atrial fibrillation

C. Elevated LVEDP with normal left atrial (LA) pressure

D. Elevated LVEDP with high LA pressure

314. This patient has:

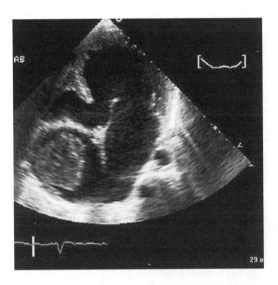

A. Tricuspid atresia

B. Right atrial myxoma

C. Hydatid cyst of the heart

D. Hypoplastic left heart syndrome

315. The flow shown here is consistent with:

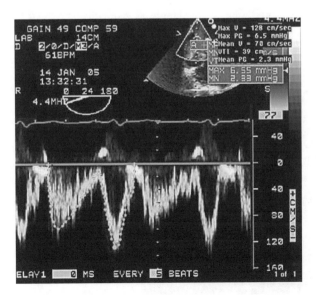

A. Superior vena cava (SVC) flow

B. Pulmonary vein flow

C. Atrial septal defect (ASD) flow

D. None of the above

316. This patient had secundum ASD fairly circular with a diameter of 2 cm. The heart rate was 61/min. The approximate shunt flow would be:

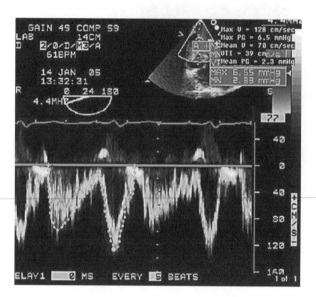

A. 5 L/min

B. 7.4 L/min

C. 13 L/min

D. 20 L/min

317. The abnormality shown in this image could be associated with:

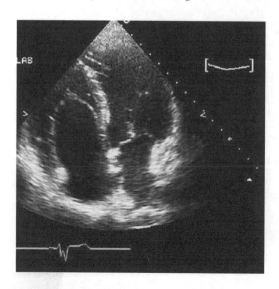

A. Accessory pathway
B. Atrial septal defect
C. Tricuspid regurgitation
D. All of the above

318. The patient shown here has:

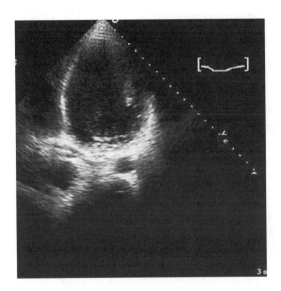

A. Prosthetic mitral valve
B. Tricuspid atresia
C. Left SVC
D. Biventricular pacemaker

319. The cause of the abnormality shown here could be due to:

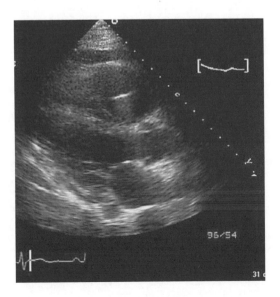

    A. Persistent left SVC

    B. Congestive heart failure

    C. Unroofed coronary sinus

    D. All of the above

320. The patient shown here has:

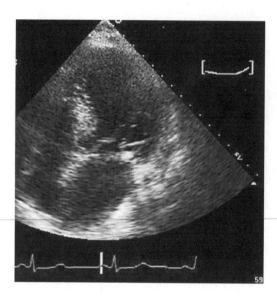

    A. Severe mitral annular calcification

    B. Mitral annuloplasty ring

    C. Rheumatic mitral valve disease

    D. None of the above

Answers for chapter 16

301. **Answer: D.**

   Posterior mitral annuloplasty ring in cross-section. This is circular in cross-section and on the atrial side of the base of the posterior mitral leaflet. Mitral annular calcification on the contrary will bury the leaflet base inside the calcification and generally starts from the base of the annulus and extends to the leaflets, and the shape is not circular in cross-section. There is no restriction of the leaflet tips to suggest rheumatic involvement and SAM is evaluated in systole. This is a diastolic frame.

302. **Answer: B.**

   This is a signal originating from A–V valve regurgitation as it starts with the QRS without any isovolumic contraction. Accompanying forward flow velocity is less than ½ m/s suggesting tricuspid origin. Mitral inflow velocity tends to be higher. The velocity of this signal is 3.2 m/s resulting in a transvalvular gradient of about 40 mmHg. Assuming an RA pressure of 10 mmHg, the RV systolic pressure would be 50 mmHg. Aortic signal is of shorter duration and starts later after the isovolumic contraction period and if mitral inflow is visible the isovolumic relaxation time could be discerned, i.e. the aortic velocity curve will not be continuous with the mitral inflow velocity curve. In acute severe MR the gradient could be low due to hypotension and high LA pressure. In such a situation a large V wave would result in rapid deceleration of the signal soon after finishing acceleration. This is so-called V wave "cutoff" sign.

303. **Answer: B.**

   End diastolic pulmonary regurgitation velocity is 2 m/s, consistent with a PA to right ventricular (RV) end diastolic gradient of 16 mmHg (4×2^2), and assuming the RV end diastolic pressure is close to the mean RA pressure the PA diastolic pressure will be 26 mmHg.

304. **Answer: C.**

   Number 1 indicates pericardial effusion, 2 indicates pleural effusion and 3 is the descending aorta. Pericardial effusion is always anterior to the aorta and pleural effusion extends posteriorly. The structure separating the two is combined parietal pericardium and pleura. The combined thickness is <3 mm, which is normal.

305. **Answer: D.**

   There is reduced aortic valve opening with every third beat. This is due to reduced transaortic flow with every third beat, which is assisted by the LVAD, and the bulk of the cardiac output is delivered through the assist device. During the intervening two beats all the stroke volume is delivered through the aortic valve. With 1:3 IABP support the increase in stroke volume during the IABP deflation occurs through the aortic valve, hence there is increased opening. In pulsus alternans, strong and weak beats alternate in 1:2 fashion. In HOCM mid-systolic closure occurs with every beat.

306. **Answer: C.**

   Echodense walls and echoluscent lumen of the cannula are seen. This LVAD cannula serves to deliver blood to the assist device. In these patients it is important to make sure that there is no obstruction to the inlet cannula by surrounding structures, including the ventricular septum, and no apical thrombi. Thrombus does not have a central luscency. False tendons are echodense and linear and rib artifacts are lighter and generally go through the anatomic boundaries.

307. **Answer: A.**

This vessel is posterior to the left atrium, indicative of descending thoracic aorta. Coronary sinus is in the posterior A–V groove and is intrapericardial. The left PA and the left lower pulmonary vein are far away from this location.

308. **Answer: A.**

An LV apical thrombus. There is a distinctly demarcated thrombus in the apex. When there is a question this can be confirmed by obtaining additional views of the apex, such as two-chamber and short axis views. Color flow imaging is at a low Nyquist limit and uses transpulmonary contrast agents such as Definity. Thrombus will be seen as a filling defect. The LV apex is a common place for a false tendon and may be mistaken for a thrombus. Rib artifact is less dense, goes beyond the endocardium and does not move with the heart.

309. **Answer: A.**

Heart failure. Dilated inferior vena cava (IVC) is suggestive of high RA pressure if it does not collapse with inspiration. Occasionally in normal young individuals one may see a dilated IVC, which readily collapses with inspiration. A general guideline is that IVC >2 cm and <10% collapse indicates RA pressure >20 mmHg, >2 cm and 50% collapse indicates RA pressure of 15 mmHg, 1.5–2 cm and > 50% collapse indicates RA pressure of 10 mmHg and <1 cm and >50% collapse indicates RA pressure of 5 mmHg.

310. **Answer: B.**

Mixed aortic valve disease with significant AS and AR. Diastolic signal is diagnostic of AR with a 4 m/s early diastolic velocity, which does not occur with MS. The velocity curve of AR is continuous with the systolic signal, indicating signal origin at the same valve. The MR signal would have a longer signal and overlap both the initial and terminal portions of the AR signal, as MR would occur with both isovolumic contraction and relaxation phases. Typical VSD signal will have a systolic component and a presystolic associated with left atrial contraction directed into the RV. If the patient has Eisenmenger's syndrome the flow velocity would be very low.

311. **Answer: D.**

All of the above. The AR signal decelerates rapidly with a pressure half-time of 185 ms (less than 250 ms indicates very rapid deceleration). The end diastolic velocity is about 2 ms, indicating an end diastolic gradient between the aorta and LV of 16 mmHg, assuming alignment of the ultrasound beam parallel to flow. As the patient's diastolic pressure is 65 mmHg, the LVEDP is 49 mmHg (65−16). Severe AR, generally acute or significant AR in the presence of stiff LV, may occur with severe AS or hypertension; high LVEDP resulting from this may cause diastolic MR and presystolic closure of the mitral valve.

312. **Answer: A.**

Severe valvular AS. The timing of the onset slightly after the onset of the QRS complex, suggestive of onset after the LV isovolumic contraction period, is suggestive of aortic origin. Though the aortic valve area is the best indicator of AS severity, a mean gradient of >50 mmHg is generally consistent with severe AS. In addition the signal is mid to late peaking, which has the same significance as the mid to late peaking of the AS murmur. SAM would cause a dagger-shaped, late peaking signal because of the dynamic nature of the obstruction.

313. **Answer: D.**

Elevated LVEDP with high LA pressure. The D-wave velocity, which is higher than the S-wave velocity with a rapid deceleration (time < 170 ms), is indicative of high LA pressure in an adult. This pattern could be normal in children because of very efficient LV relaxation. In the example shown here the AR wave duration is markedly increased. Normally AR wave duration is less than mitral A-wave duration and is less than 110–120 ms. Though A-wave duration is not shown here, the AR wave duration is grossly abnormal at 200 ms, indicating high LVEDP and causing an increase in the duration of atrial systole because of increased atrial afterload. In a volume-depleted patient the S wave will be prominent and the AR wave would be diminutive; in atrial fibrillation the AR wave is lost.

314. **Answer: A.**

Tricuspid atresia. The image shows an absent tricuspid valve, a right atrial mass that is consistent and likely to be a thrombus due to stasis and a ventricular septal defect. This patient had cavopulmonary anastomosis with SVC–RPA and RA–LPA shunt such that IVC blood drained into the LPA through the RA, causing thrombus formation. The PA was completely banded to facilitate cavopulmonary flow. This patient has a well-developed left heart and hence does not have hypoplastic left heart syndrome. Right atrial myxoma is a possibility but thrombus is much more likely in this situation.

315. **Answer: C.**

ASD flow. The flow shown is typical of ASD flow with systolic–diastolic wave and a second wave associated with atrial contraction, all left to right in the same direction. Both SVC and pulmonary vein flows are triphasic with S, D and AR waves, with the AR wave being in an opposite direction to S and D waves.

316. **Answer: B.**

7.4 L/min. The shunt flow per heart beat is the time velocity integral (TVI) across the defect × cross sectional area, i.e. $39 \times 3.14 = 122$ cc. Shunt flow per minute = shunt volume per beat × heart rate = $122 \times 61 = 7.4$ L/min.

317. **Answer: D.**

The image is diagnostic of Epstein's anomaly of the tricuspid valve. This is diagnosed when the attachment of the septal leaflet of the tricuspid valve is apically displaced in relation to the anterior mitral leaflet by >8 mm. In this disorder the septal leaflet is large, sail-like and could be plastered to the RV wall through the chordae tendinae. The associations include severe tricuspid regurgitation, atrial septal defect and right-sided accessory pathway causing PSVT.

318. **Answer: D.**

Biventricular pacemaker. A coronary sinus lead is clearly seen in this image. This is imaged from the apical four-chamber view with a posterior transducer tilt to obtain a tomographic plane through the coronary sinus. Because of this the mitral valve is not seen. The coronary sinus is not enlarged to support the diagnosis of left SVC.

319. **Answer: D.**

All of the above. The coronary sinus is dilated, which could be due to increased flow or pressure and any of the conditions listed can potentially result in a dilated coronary sinus. Note that the coronary sinus is in the A–V groove and intrapericardial versus descending aorta, which is in the posterior mediastinum and is extrapericardial.

320. **Answer: B.**

Mitral annuloplasty ring. Echocardiographically this is distinguished from mitral annular calcification by its rounded shape in cross-section and projection into the left atrium at the base of the posterior leaflet. On the contrary mitral annular calcification would incorporate the base of the posterior mitral leaflet into itself.

Chapter 17

321. The cause of dyspnea in this patient is likely to be due to:

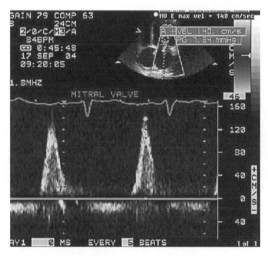

   A. Left heart failure
   B. Primary pulmonary hypertension
   C. Chronic obstructive pulmonary disorder
   D. None of the above

322. This is an end systolic frame in a patient with shortness of breath. The most likely diagnosis is:

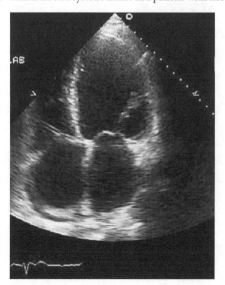

    A. Ebstein's anomaly

    B. Hypertrophic cardiomyopathy

    C. Atrial septal defect

    D. Dilated cardiomyopathy

323. The most likely mechanism of mitral regurgitation (MR) in this patient is:

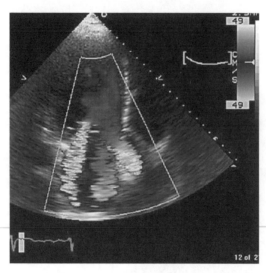

    A. P2 tethering

    B. P2 prolapse

    C. Bileaflet mitral valve prolapse

    D. None of the above

    (There is a full-colour version of this image in the colour plate section of this book)

324. This 19-year-old patient was stabbed in the precordial area. Examination revealed a loud systolic murmur. The most likely cause of this murmur is:

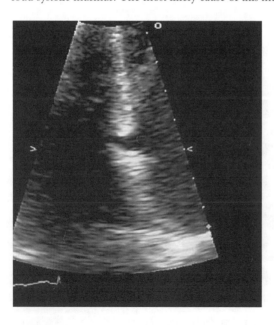

A. Penetrating injury to the interventricular septum

B. Mitral valve prolapse

C. Hypertrophic obstructive cardiomyopathy (HOCM)

D. None of the above

325. This trans–esophageal echocardiogram (TEE) image is obtained from the upper esophagus and the aortic arch is shown on the top. The arrow points to:

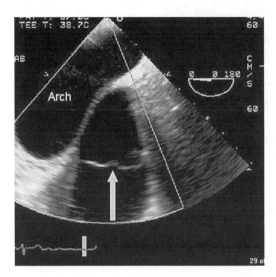

A. Pulmonary valve

B. Aortic valve

C. Mitral valve

D. Tricuspid valve

326. The structure indicated by the arrow is:

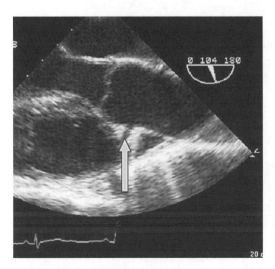

A. Right coronary artery (RCA)

B. Left coronary artery (LCA)

C. Entry tear into dissection

D. None of the above

327. This is a suprasternal image of the aortic arch, suggestive of:

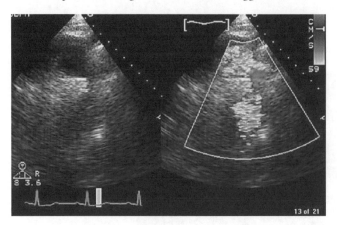

A. Coarctation of the aorta

B. Severe aortic regurgitation (AR)

C. Patent ductus arteriosus (PDA)

D. None of the above

(There is a full-colour version of this image in the colour plate section of this book)

328. In the accompanying image the structure indicated by the arrow is:

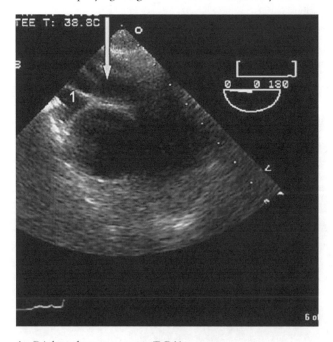

A. Right pulmonary artery (RPA)

B. Left atrium

C. Aortic arch

D. Right upper pulmonary vein

329. The structure denoted by the arrow is:

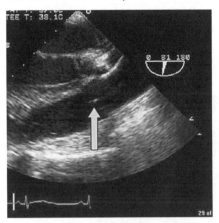

    A. An artifact
    B. Pulmonary valve
    C. Aortic valve
    D. Subpulmonic stenosis

330. What is the abnormality in the accompanying image:

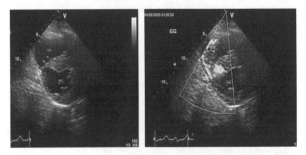

    A. Congenital muscular ventricular septal defect (VSD)
    B. Post-infarction posterior VSD
    C. Artifact of the normal posterior thinning at the valve plane
    D. Post-myectomy of HOCM

    (There is a full-colour version of this image in the colour plate section of this book)

331. The abnormal finding in this image is:

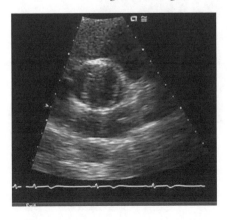

A. Bicuspid aortic valve

B. Aortic dissection flap

C. Aortic aneurysm

D. None of the above

332. Mitral regurgitation (MR) signal shown here is suggestive of:

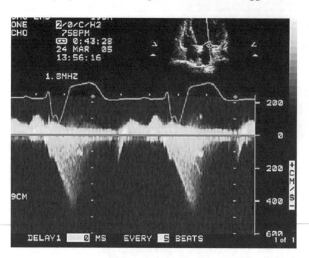

A. Some diastolic MR in addition to systolic MR

B. Markedly depressed left ventricular (LV) dp/dt

C. Both

D. Neither

333. Mitral flow profile shown here is suggestive of:

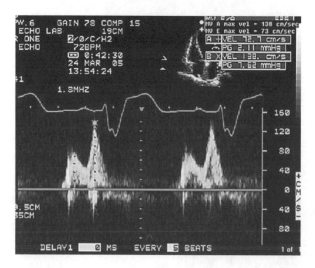

A. Normal LV diastolic function

B. Abnormal relaxation

C. Pseudonormal pattern

D. Restrictive pattern

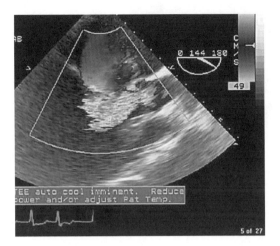

A. Normal flow in the left ventricular outflow tract (LVOT)

B. Subvalvular aortic stenosis (AS)

C. Aortic regurgitation

D. None of the above

(There is a full-colour version of this image in the colour plate section of this book)

335. This continuous wave Doppler signal is suggestive of:

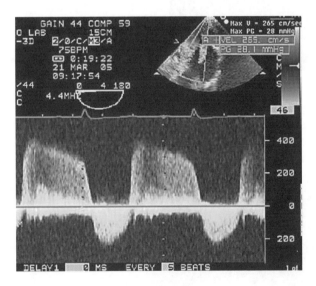

A. AS and AR

B. Mitral stenosis (MS) and MR

C. VSD flow

D. Aortic flow in a patient with coarctation

336. This continuous wave signal obtained from the mid-trans-esophageal location is indicative of:

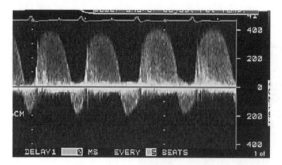

A. AS and AR

B. MS and MR

C. VSD flow

D. None of the above

337. This is a TEE image from the mid–esophagus of a late diastolic frame of the aortic valve: This patient is most likely to have:

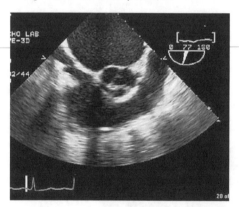

A. Severe aortic regurgitation

B. Severe aortic stenosis

C. HOCM

D. Ascending aortic dissection

338. This patient is most likely to have:

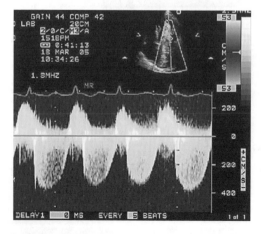

A. Acute severe MR

B. Chronic severe MR

C. Severe MS and mild MR

D. None of the above

339. This patient had *Staphylococcus aureus* endocarditis of the aortic valve. The most likely cause is:

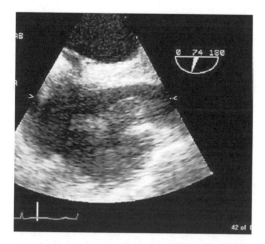

A. Central venous catheter–associated infection

B. Dental work

C. Immunosuppressed state

D. Intravenous drug use

340. The image of the aortic valve is suggestive of :

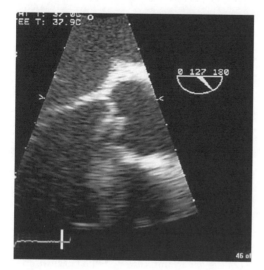

A. Aortic valve vegetation

B. Node of Arantius

C. Lambl's excrescences

D. Ascending aortic dissection causing prolapse of the noncoronary cusp

Answers for chapter 17

321. **Answer: A.**

Left heart failure. The mitral inflow shown here is indicative of high left atrial (LA) pressure. Though the patient is in atrial fibrillation with only E wave, the E wave deceleration is very rapid.

322. **Answer: D.**

Dilated cardiomyopathy. There is a four-chamber dilatation. There is no increase in wall thickness to suggest HOCM. In atrial septal defect both the right ventricle and the right atrium will be dilated due to volume overload with normal LA and LV size. The tricuspid valve position is normal and hence does not support the diagnosis of Ebstein's anomaly.

323. **Answer: A.**

P2 tethering. This is an apical long axis view, showing A2 and P2 scallops of the mitral valve. The MR jet is directed posterolaterally towards P2, consistent with P2 tethering. A similar jet direction can also occur in A2 prolapse, but both leaflets coapt distal to the plane of mitral annulus. Bileaflet prolapse of equal magnitude will result in a central jet.

324. **Answer: A.**

Penetrating injury to the interventricular septum. A defect is seen in the ventricular septum. This patient had a penetrating injury to the septum. The image does not support the presence of mitral valve prolapse or hypertrophic septum.

325. **Answer: A.**

Pulmonary valve. Pulmonary valve and the main pulmonary artery are seen. This is a good view to examine these structures and also to obtain spectral Doppler signals from the pulmonary valve and pulmonary artery.

326. **Answer: A.**

Right coronary artery. This is the classical location of the RCA. The LCA is not seen in the aortic long axis view. Because of its left lateral location it is seen in the short axis view. There is no aortic dissection and entry tear into dissection would be a hole in the endothelium and is not tubular in shape.

327. **Answer: A.**

Coarctation of the aorta. Narrowing and turbulence at the junction of the arch and descending aorta are clearly seen, indicative of coarctation. In severe AR, flow reversal is holodiastolic. There is no communication between the aorta and the pulmonary artery, suggestive of PDA.

328. **Answer: A.**

Right pulmonary artery. This is a TEE image from the proximal esophageal location, a high basal view above the level of the left atrium. Also note the linear shadows in the RPA, which are commonly seen and represent mirror image artifacts. A short axis image of the RPA or color flow image at a low scale would confirm this. The large circular structure is the ascending aorta and number 1 is the SVC in cross-section. Also note the reverberations from a catheter in the SVC.

329. **Answer: B.**

Pulmonary valve. This is a TEE image from mid- to low-esophageal location showing the long axis of the pulmonary valve and the proximal pulmonary artery. The RVOT is clearly seen as well.

330. **Answer: B.**

Post-infarction posterior VSD. There is marked thinning of the mid-inferior wall and inferior septum without any scarring. There is also a defect establishing communication between the LV and the RV and the color flow confirms this. This is classical post-infarct posterior VSD and a short axis view of the LV at all levels would help to delineate the pathology. Such thinning does not occur in congenital VSD. The location of iatrogenic infarct or myectomy in HOCM is in the proximal anterior septum.

331. **Answer: A.**

Bicuspid aortic valve. This is a classic bicuspid aortic valve. Though a dissection flap in a patient with circumferential dissection with a central true lumen may mimic this, both leaflets and commissures are clearly seen here. This image is at the level of the aortic annulus and the rest of the ascending aorta is not shown to comment about nondissecting aortic aneurysm.

332. **Answer: C.**

Both. The initial portion of the signal at low velocity represents diastolic MR, which occurs during left atrial relaxation and may be due to a long PR interval or high left ventricular end diastolic pressure (LVEDP). The rate of velocity rise of the MR signal is very slow. The normal time taken for the MR velocity to increase from 1 to 3 m/s is 10–20 ms, representing an LV dp/dt of 1600–3200 mmHg/s. In this example this interval is 160 ms, giving an average rate of pressure rise during early systole (loosely called LV dp/dt and correlates with this) is 200 mmHg/s. Also note the very prolonged QRS duration. The main determinants of LV dp/dt include LV contractility, heart rate, preload and LV systolic synchrony, which would be abnormal in left bundle branch block.

333. **Answer: B.**

Abnormal relaxation. Suggested by an E/A ratio of <1. Though the E-wave deceleration time is <250 ms, generally the isovolumic relaxation time (not shown here) tends to be greater than 100 ms. The E/A ratio can be lower in the elderly because of age-related LV relaxation failure, patients with low filling pressures, more rapid heart rates and those with prolongation of the PR interval. In a pseudonormal pattern the mitral inflow looks normal, but there is some other evidence of LV relaxation abnormality, such as reduced Em velocity, reduced mitral flow propagation or increased duration of atrial systole as judged by pulmonary vein flow (AR wave reversal duration). Restrictive pattern is characterized by an E/A ratio of >2, E-wave deceleration of <150 ms and isovolumic relaxation time duration of <70 ms.

334. **Answer: C.**

Aortic regurgitation. Note the diastolic frame showing an AR jet.

335. **Answer: A.**

AS and AR. Unlike the MR signal, the AS signal occupies only the ejection period and is absent during the isovolumic contraction time. Hence the signal starts a few milliseconds after the QRS. The diastolic velocity is too high for MS. This order of gradient and LA pressure would be incompatible with life. VSD flow is predominantly systolic with a presystolic component caused by atrial contraction. The gradient across a coarctation is systolic, the duration increases with greater degrees of stenosis and there may be a diastolic gradient. However both the systolic and diastolic components will be in the same direction.

336. **Answer: B.**

MS and MR. Please see explanation to question 335.

337. **Answer: A.**

Severe aortic regurgitation. The aortic leaflets are thickened with rolled-up edges and a central coaptation defect in end diastole. This anatomy would be associated with wide-open aortic regurgitation, as the regurgitant orifice is visible by anatomic imaging. Aortic stenosis cannot be diagnosed by a diastolic frame. HOCM typically causes mid-systolic closure of the aortic valve, best visualized by M mode. Aortic dissection may cause AR by one of several mechanisms: dilatation of sino-tubular junction, leaflet tethering, extension of hematoma into the aortic leaflet causing it to prolapse, or as a result of the primary problem such as bicuspid aortic valve or annulo-aortic ectasia.

338. **Answer: C.**

Chronic severe MR. The MR signal density is more than 60% of the mitral inflow signal. This correlates with a volume of regurgitation. In addition, the mitral inflow velocity is increased without a slow deceleration. A slow deceleration would indicate significant mitral stenosis. Despite severe MR, the profile of the MR signal is quite rounded without the rapid deceleration that would typically be seen in acute severe MR, because of the large left atrial V wave, the so-called "V wave cutoff sign".

339. **Answer: A.**

Central venous catheter-associated infection. This bicaval trans-esophageal view shows a large mass in the superior vena cava, which is typically associated with a central catheter-associated thrombus or vegetation. This most likely is the cause of his sepsis and endocarditis. In addition there is a possible defect at the superior portion of the fossa ovalis, suggesting a patent foramen ovale (PFO). This patient had a large PFO by color and contrast echocardiography, allowing paradoxical embolization of the bacterial mass to cause left-sided endocarditis, escaping the protective filtration mechanism offered by the lung.

340. **Answer: A.**

Aortic valve vegetation. The mass on the aortic valve is suggestive of mass on the left ventricular side of the aortic valve. This is suggestive of vegetation. Also, there is prolapse of the noncoronary cusp, causing significant AR, and this is due to leaflet destruction with endocarditis. The other mechanism for prolapse could be a bicuspid aortic valve with prolapse of the larger cusp. Node of Arantius, as the name suggests, is a nodular thickening of the central portion of the leaflet edge and is best visualized from the short axis view of the valve. Lambl's excrescences are thin filamentous structures attached to the leaflet margin. There is no evidence of aortic dissection or intramural hematoma in this patient.

Chapter 18

Questions

341. This continuous wave Doppler signal is indicative of:

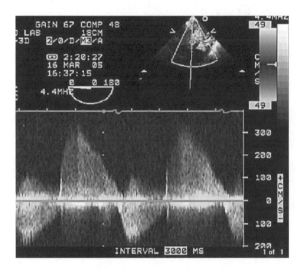

A. Acute severe aortic regurgitation (AR)
B. Chronic compensated AR
C. Severe aortic stenosis (AS)
D. Severe mixed mitral valve disease

342. This trans–esophageal echocardiogram (TEE) image is suggestive of:

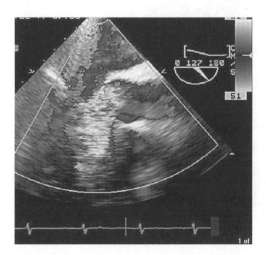

A. Severe AR

B. Hypertrophic obstructive cardiomyopathy (HOCM)

C. Subaortic membranous aortic stenosis

D. None of the above

(There is a full-colour version of this image in the colour plate section of this book)

343. This pulse wave Doppler flow signal in the descending thoracic aorta on a TEE is indicative of:

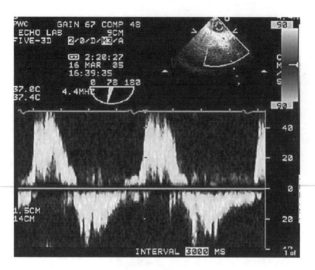

A. Coarctation of the aorta

B. Middle aortic syndrome

C. Severe AR

D. HOCM

344. What procedure did this patient undergo?

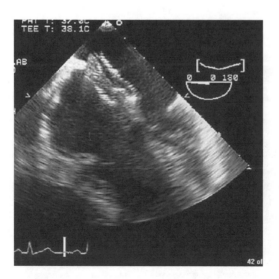

    A. Mitral valve replacement

    B. Atrial septal defect (ASD) closure with an Amplatzer device

    C. Patent foramen ovale (PFO) closure with cardioseal device

    D. Closure of ASD with a pericardial patch

345. This patient is likely to have:

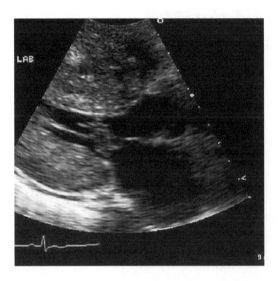

    A. Systolic murmur accentuated by Valsalva maneuver

    B. Early peaking systolic murmur

    C. Early diastolic murmur heard in sitting position at end expiration

    D. A mid-diastolic murmur best heard with the bell in left lateral position

346. This signal shown here is likely to be caused by:

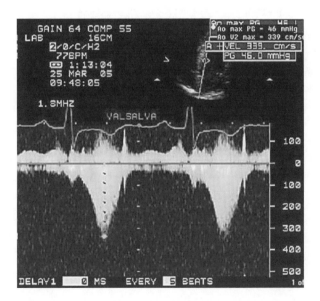

    A. HOCM

    B. Critical valvular aortic stenosis

    C. Acute mitral regurgitation (MR)

    D. None of the above

347. The image shown here is suggestive of:

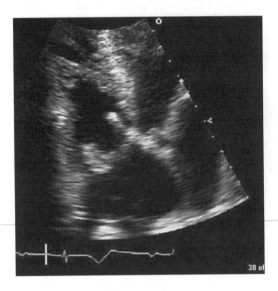

    A. Bioprosthetic tricuspid valve

    B. Carcinoid valvulopathy of tricuspid valve

    C. Tricuspid annuloplasty ring

    D. Large tricuspid vegetation

348. This 65-year-old patient with MR is likely to have:

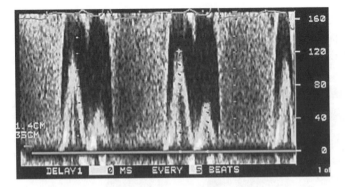

    A. An opening snap

    B. Third heart sound

    C. Fourth heart sound

    D. Summation gallop

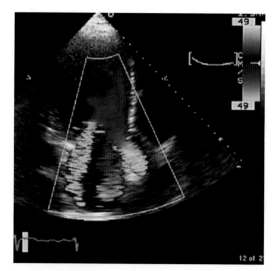

Question 323

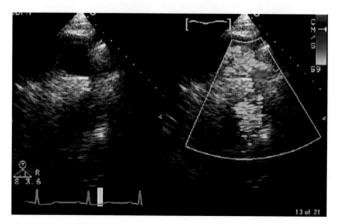

Question 327

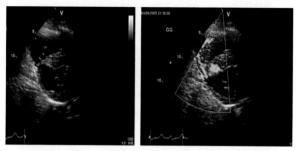

Question 330

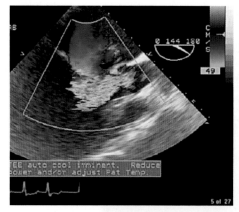

Question 334

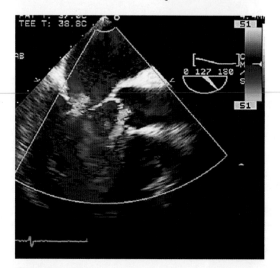

Question 342

Question 351

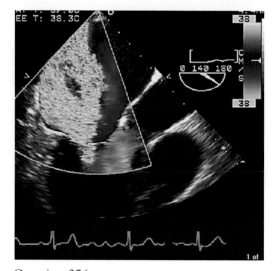

Question 356

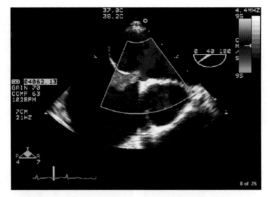

Question 362

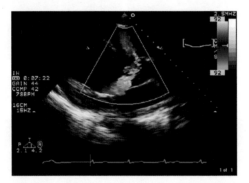

Question 363

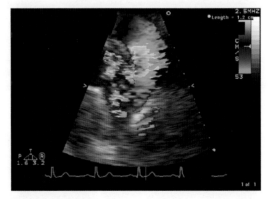

Question 373

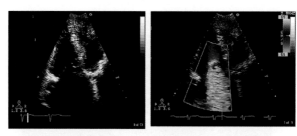

Question 376

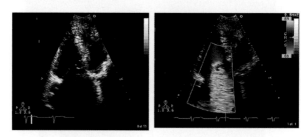

Question 377

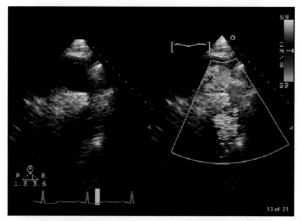

Question 394 (top image)

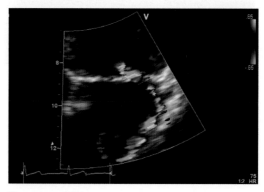

Question 397

349. The CW Doppler signal is consistent with:

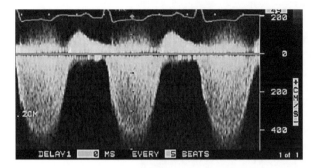

   A. Critical AS
   B. Severe MR
   C. Maladie de Roger
   D. None of the above

350. This tricuspid regurgitation (TR) signal was obtained from TEE. The clinically estimated right atrial (RA) pressure in this patient was 20 mmHg and there is no pulmonary stenosis. The pulmonary artery (PA) systolic pressure in this patient would be:

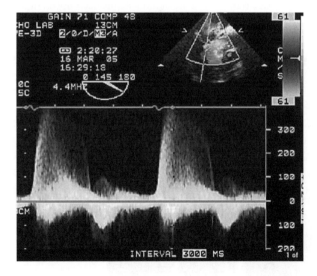

   A. 30 mmHg
   B. 50 mmHg
   C. 70 mmHg
   D. Cannot be calculated

351. This patient is likely to have:

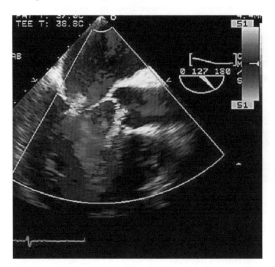

    A. Acute severe AR
    B. Mild AR
    C. Mitral stenosis
    D. None of the above
    (There is a full-colour version of this image in the colour plate section of this book)

352. This transmitral flow is obtained from the esophageal transducer location from a patient with *Staphylococcus aureus* bacteremia and acute hemodynamic decompensation. Patient is in sinus rhythm. The most likely cause of his decompensation is:

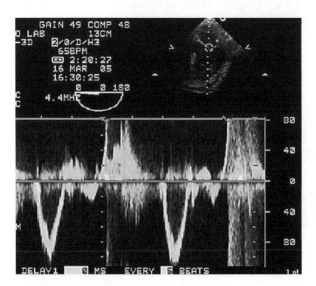

    A. Acute MR
    B. Acute AR
    C. Rupture of the ventricular septum
    D. None of the above

353. The cause of this patient's multiple bilateral lung abscesses is:

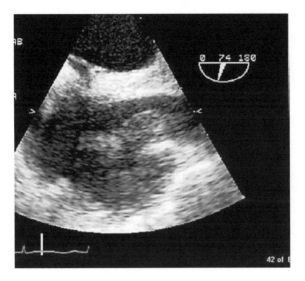

    A. Vegetation in superior vena cava (SVC)
    B. Tricuspid endocarditis
    C. Probable immune deficiency; no vegetation seen on image shown
    D. None of the above

354. The cause of heart failure in this 30-year-old man is likely to be:

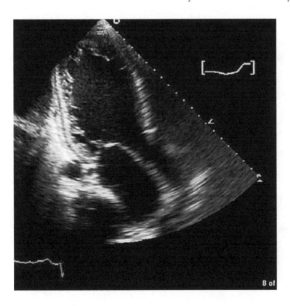

    A. Noncompaction of the left ventricle (LV)
    B. Hemochromatosis
    C. Cardiac amyloid
    D. Hypertrophic cardiomyopathy

355. The structure indicated by the arrow is:

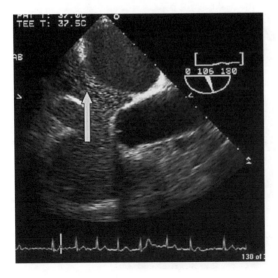

A. Inferior vena cava (IVC)–RA junction

B. Superior vena cava

C. Anomalously draining right upper pulmonary vein

D. Atrial septal defect

356. The MR flow rate in this patient (PISA radius of 0.9 cm, aliasing velocity of 38 cm/sec) is approximately:

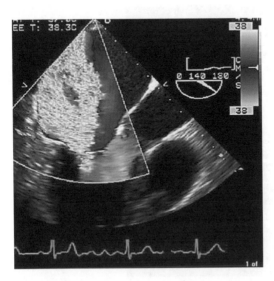

A. 200 cc/s

B. 200 cc/min

C. 100 cc/min

D. 100 cc/s

(There is a full-colour version of this image in the colour plate section of this book)

357. The patient shown is likely to have:

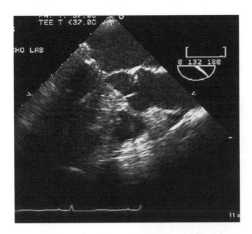

A. An early diastolic murmur
B. Late peaking systolic ejection murmur with absent A2 component of S2
C. Late peaking systolic murmur increased by Valsalva's maneuver and normal A2
D. Mid-diastolic murmur

358. The most likely diagnosis in this patient is:

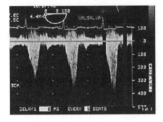 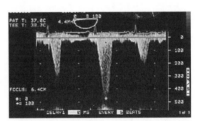

At rest   **With Valsalva**

A. HOCM
B. Severe aortic stenosis
C. Mitral valve prolapse
D. None of the above

359. This patient is likely to have:

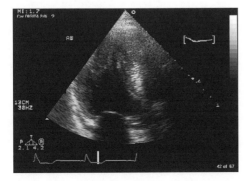

A. Apical HOCM

B. Hypertensive heart disease

C. Endomyocardial fibrosis

D. None of the above

360. The appearance of the atrial septum in this patient is due to:

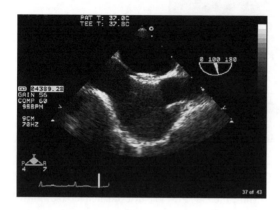

A. ASD repair with a pericardial patch

B. ASD closure device

C. PFO closure device

D. None of the above

Answers for chapter 18

341. **Answer: A.**

Acute severe AR. There is a rapid deceleration of the AR profile indicating rapidly diminishing aorto-left ventricular pressure gradient, which is typically seen in acute severe AR, mostly due to rapid rise in LV diastolic pressure, due to regurgitation in a noncompliant nonconditioned left ventricle. It is also possible to get this in a chronic severe AR, with severe vasodilatation, which would cause a low aortic diastolic pressure, but this scenario is less frequent. The systolic signal is early peaking, with a velocity of only 2 m/s, with severe AR indicating the absence of any significant AS. The onset of the systolic signal after the isovolumic contraction period indicates its origin at the semilunar valve as opposed to origin at the A–V valve. This systolic velocity is too low for MR unless the continuous wave signal is malaligned to the MR jet direction; this is unlikely as the signal is not bidirectional and the diastolic velocity is too high for MS.

342. **Answer: A.**

Severe aortic regurgitation. This diastolic frame is indicated by the open mitral valve and the left ventricular outflow tract (LVOT) is completely filled with turbulent flow typical of wide-open aortic regurgitation. Note that this is not a systolic frame to indicate subvalvular aortic stenosis.

343. **Answer: C.**

Severe aortic regurgitation. A prominent holodiastolic flow reversal suggesting retrograde flow in the aorta is seen. This flow would also cause Duroziez's murmur by physical exam due to the turbulence produced by partial occlusion by the finger, which would produce a diastolic murmur in the proximal femoral artery. Coarctation and middle aortic syndrome diminish pulsatility in the distal aortic flow and the flow becomes continuous due to flow through collaterals. Though HOCM can produce mid-systolic closure of the aortic valve, it does not produce any flow disturbance in the distal aorta.

344. **Answer: B.**

ASD closure with Amplatzer. This is a typical appearance of an Amplatzer device. Both the left and right atrial discs are seen, sandwiching the atrial septum. The role of TEE during ASD closure includes sizing of the defect, with and without balloon inflation, examination of adequacy of rims, ruling out anomalous pulmonary venous connections, guiding deployment and ascertaining post deployment lack of impingement into SVC, right upper pulmonary vein, IVC and the mitral valve, in addition to excluding any residual ASD. Small flow through the device is normal, until it becomes endothelialized.

345. **Answer: A.**

Systolic murmur accentuated by Valsalva's maneuver. This is a mid-systolic frame showing systolic anterior motion (SAM) of the anterior mitral leaflet. As SAM increases in late systole the gradient will be maximal in end systole, causing a late peaking systolic murmur. Both the gradient and murmur are increased by Valsalva's maneuver through a diminution of LV volume, causing an increase in SAM. Early diastolic murmur heard in the sitting position at end expiration is typical of aortic regurgitation. A mid-diastolic murmur best heard with the bell in the left lateral position is typical of mitral stenosis.

346. **Answer: A.**

HOCM. This late peaking dagger-shaped signal is typical of SAM caused by HOCM. This occurs due to the dynamic LVOT obstruction increases through systole. Critical valvular AS is unlikely as in this case the velocity is likely to be higher (unless cardiac output is very low) and the signal contour would be more rounded. Acute MR gives rise to an early peaking signal with a rapid deceleration because of a large left atrial V wave, the so-called V wave cut-off sign. In LV cavity obliteration this signal will be much later peaking, with a gradient only in the very late part of systole when there is very little blood left in the distal LV cavity.

347. **Answer: A.**

Bioprosthetic tricuspid valve. This patient has Hancock porcine bioprosthetic tricuspid valve. The struts of the bioprosthetic valve are well seen. An annuloplasty ring would be seen as a small rounded structure in cross-section at the tricuspid annulus only.

348. **Answer: B.**

Third heart sound. The mitral inflow is suggestive of high left atrial pressure. The mitral E/A ratio is >2 and deceleration time is 60 ms, indicating very high left atrial pressure. The calculated E-wave deceleration calculated from the E-wave amplitude and its time (velocity/time) is about 20 m/s^2. A rate of deceleration of >8–9 m/s^2 is likely to result in S3. Age is relevant, as such a filling pattern in young children is normal because they have extremely efficient LV relaxation, which would result in physiological S3. S4 results from a prominent atrial-filling wave in a stiff ventricle, and in a summation gallop the E and A waves are fused. This patient has no mitral stenosis and hence opening snap is unlikely.

349. **Answer: B.**

Severe MR. The temporal continuity of the systolic signal with the inflow signal suggests its origin at the mitral valve. The AS signal would occupy only the ejection period, being separated from the mitral inflow signal by isovolumic contraction and relaxation periods. A small ventricular septal defect (VSD) may result in a holosystolic signal, but generally has a presystolic component associated with left atrial systole, and generally this flow is directed towards the transducer from most of the imaging windows.

350. **Answer: C.**

70 mmHg. The TR velocity is 3.5 m/s, yielding an RV–RA systolic gradient of 50 mmHg. With an RA pressure of 20 mmHg the RV systolic pressure would be 70 mmHg, which would be the same as the PA systolic pressure in the absence of significant pulmonic stenosis.

351. **Answer: A.**

Acute severe aortic regurgitation. This late diastolic frame shows diastolic mitral regurgitation. There is also aortic regurgitation by color. The mitral valve is closed prematurely. This combination of findings is consistent with acute severe aortic regurgitation. A smaller AR jet in late diastole was due to late diastolic equilibration of aortic and left ventricular pressures. Diastolic MR results from the receipt of AR volume in an LV with high operating end diastolic stiffness.

352. **Answer: B.**

Acute aortic regurgitation. The Doppler flow suggests premature closure of the mitral valve with lack of A wave despite being in sinus rhythm. This is pathognomonic of acute AR causing rapidly rising LV diastolic pressure due to failure to accommodate a large acute volume overload. In acute AR the left atrium would still be contracting, but would be unable to eject against an acute increase in afterload. Pulmonary vein flow profile in this patient would show a prominent AR wave and the tricuspid inflow would still have the A wave. Acute MR and VSD would not eliminate the A wave unless the patient had a recent episode of atrial fibrillation and the atrium is stunned.

353. **Answer: A.**

Vegetation in superior vena cava. The image shows large vegetation protruding into the right atrium. This was catheter related causing *Staphylococcus* bacteremia. Imaging the whole length of the SVC, right atrial endocardium and the Eustachian valve is extremely important in patients with central catheters or PICC lines with fever or suspected bacteremia.

354. **Answer: A.**

Noncompaction of the left ventricle. The inferolateral wall of the LV in this patient is heavily trabeculated; noncompacted (trabeculated) to compacted wall thickness ratio is more than 2:1. This is highly indicative of noncompaction of LV myocardium, which is a developmental disorder causing congestive heart failure. In the other three conditions the LV myocardium would be thicker, either due to infiltration or increased myocardial mass.

355. **Answer: A.**

Inferior vena cava–right atrium junction. Part of proximal IVC is seen with entry of saline contrast, in the longitudinal plane from a TEE. With this orientation caudal structures are seen on the left and cephalad structures are seen on the right. This patient has a prominent Eustachian valve, and in a patient with a prominent Eustachian valve, in a low esophageal view, where left atrium is not seen, this junction may be mistaken for an atrial septal defect. This patient was referred from an outside facility with that mistaken diagnosis from a TEE.

356. **Answer: A.**

200 cc/s. The regurgitant flow rate equals $2\pi r^2 \times$ Nyquist limit. Here the proximal isovelocity surface area (PISA) radius is 0.9 cm and the Nyquist limit is 38 cm/s. Regurgitant flow rate $= 6.28 \times 0.9 \times 0.9 \times 38 = 200$ cc/s.

357. **Answer: C.**

This patient clearly has systolic anterior motion of the anterior mitral leaflet causing LVOT obstruction. As the SAM increases in late systole, the gradient velocity and turbulence are more in late systole, causing a late peaking late systolic murmur. SAM is increased by LV volume reduction and vasodilatation. A2 is preserved in these patients in contrast to patients with severe aortic stenosis, who may also have late peaking systolic murmur.

358. **Answer: A.**

HOCM. This patient has HOCM with dynamic LVOT obstruction caused by SAM, which causes a late peaking systolic gradient, increased by Valsalva's maneuver and amyl nitrate inhalation. The gradient would also be increased by positive inotropic agents and vasodilators and decreased by an increase in afterload, with vasoconstrictors or handgrip. In addition to HOCM, SAM can occur in volume-depleted states with small LV cavity and also after surgical mitral valve repair in patients with long anterior and posterior leaflets, especially if a small annuloplasty ring is used.

359. **Answer: A.**

Apical HOCM. This patient has disproportionately thickened LV apical myocardium typical of apical HOCM. This results in a spade-shaped LV cavity in diastole. These patients also have giant T-wave inversions in their chest leads. In hypertensive heart disease LV hypotension is more uniformly distributed. Endomyocardial fibrosis causes apical obliteration due to endocardial thickening rather than myocardial thickening.

360. **Answer: C.**

PFO closure device. The image shows two parallel discs sandwiching the upper atrial septum. The right atrial disc is larger than the left atrial disc. This is suggestive of an Amplatzer PFO closure device. In an ASD closure device, the left atrial disc is larger than the right atrial disc. Patch repair of the septum will not show the triple-layer morphology as seen here.

Chapter 19

361. The image shows:

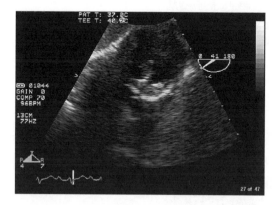

   A. Normal native tricuspid valve
   B. Normal bioprosthetic valve
   C. Vegetation on a bioprosthetic valve
   D. Avulsion of the tricuspid valve

362. This 31-year-old woman with no other medical history had two episodes of transient ischemic cerebral attacks, the first one after a long duration of air travel and the second one during straining in the rest-room. The most likely cause of this patient's attacks is:

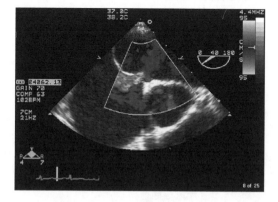

   A. Paradoxical embolism
   B. Vagally mediated atrial fibrillation
   C. Left atrial thrombus
   D. None of the above

   (There is a full-colour version of this image in the colour plate section of this book)

363. This 35-year-old patient with AIDS and bicuspid aortic valve has *Staphylococcus* bacteremia. The color flow image is suggestive of:

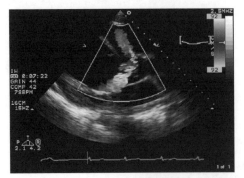

    A. Right coronary artery flow
    B. Pulmonary vegetation
    C. Fistulous communication between aorta and right ventricle (RV)
    D. None of the above
    (There is a full-colour version of this image in the colour plate section of this book)

364. This patient's bilateral *Staphylococcus* lung abscesses are likely due to:

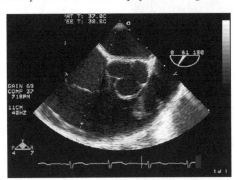

    A. Tricuspid valve endocarditis
    B. Pulmonary valve endocarditis
    C. Catheter-related infection of superior vena cava and right atrium (RA)
    D. None of the above

365. The structure indicated by the arrow is:

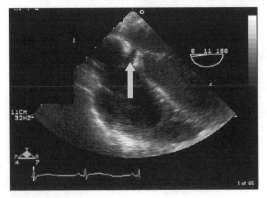

A. Coronary sinus

B. Inferior vena cava

C. Atrial septal defect

D. None of the above

366. This patient's stroke is likely due to:

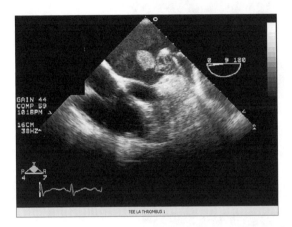

A. Left atrial thrombus

B. Left atrial myxoma

C. Mitral valve endocarditis

D. Patent foramen ovale (PFO)

367. The structure indicated by the arrow is:

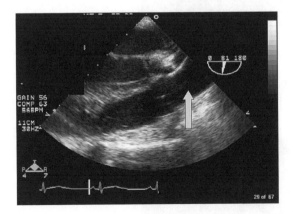

A. Main pulmonary artery (PA)

B. Ascending aorta

C. Descending aorta

D. None of the above

368. This patient with a prosthetic tricuspid valve has evidence of:

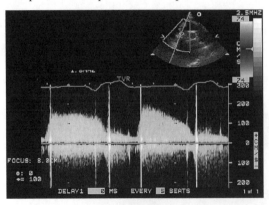

A. Normal function
B. Stenosis
C. Regurgitation
D. Endocarditis

369. The mass in the left atrium in this patient is most likely:

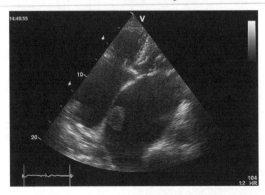

A. Thrombus
B. Myxoma
C. Metastatic lung carcinoma
D. Lipomatous septum

370. The short axis view of the heart is indicative of:

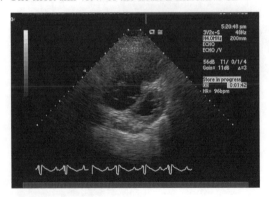

A. Severe pulmonary hypertension

B. Severe tricuspid regurgitation (TR) with normal PA pressure

C. RV infarct

D. RV dysplasia

371. The surgical procedure that this patient underwent is most likely to be:

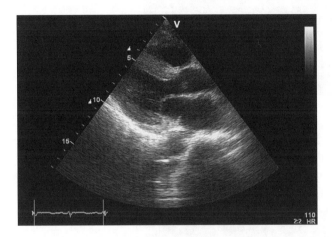

A. Orthotropic heart transplantation

B. Mitral valve repair with annuloplasty

C. Maze procedure

D. Septal myectomy for hypertrophic obstructive cardiomyopathy

372. This TR signal is from a patient with moderate TR. The most likely mechanism of TR is:

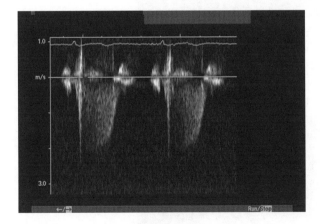

A. Pulmonary hypertension with annular dilatation

B. Flail tricuspid valve

C. Tricuspid valve prolapse

D. Cannot make a mechanistic diagnosis

373. This image of the aortic arch from the suprasternal view is suggestive of:

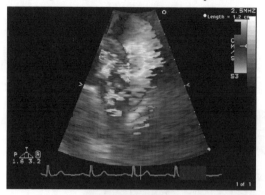

    A. Patent ductus arteriosus (PDA)

    B. Coarctation of the aorta

    C. Severe aortic regurgitation

    D. Aortic pseudoaneurysm

(There is a full-colour version of this image in the colour plate section of this book)

374. This flow velocity across the tricuspid valve is indicative of:

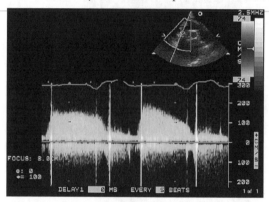

    A. Severe tricuspid stenosis

    B. Severe tricuspid regurgitation

    C. Tricuspid atresia

    D. Ebstein's anomaly

375. The TR velocity profile shown here is suggestive of:

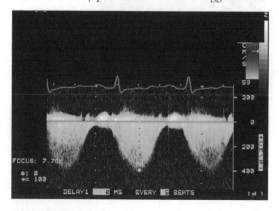

A. Normal PA pressure

B. Mild pulmonary hypertension

C. Severe pulmonary hypertension with good RV function

D. Severe pulmonary hypertension with poor RV function

376. The amount of tricuspid regurgitation in this patient is:

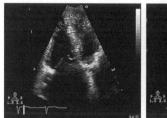
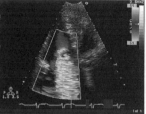

A. Mild

B. Moderate

C. Severe

D. Cannot quantify

(There is a full-colour version of this image in the colour plate section of this book)

377. The patient in question 376 is likely to have:

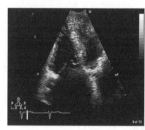
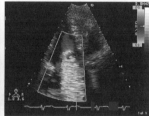

A. Normal PA pressure

B. Mild pulmonary hypertension

C. Moderate or severe pulmonary hypertension

(There is a full-colour version of this image in the colour plate section of this book)

378. The type of surgical procedure performed on this patient's mitral valve is likely to be:

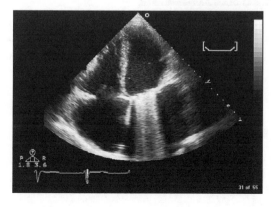

A. Mitral annuloplasty
B. Alfieri procedure
C. Replacement with a bioprosthetic valve
D. Replacement with a mechanical valve

379. What intervention can potentially change the mitral inflow pattern as shown in this image?

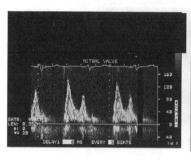 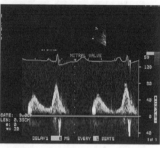

Before   After

A. Diuresis
B. Control of severe hypertension
C. Correction of severe anemia
D. All of the above

380. What is the abnormality shown here?

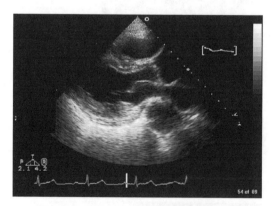

A. Thoracic aortic aneurysm
B. Cor triatriatum
C. Artifact
D. Dilated left PA

Answers for chapter 19

361. **Answer: C.**

     Vegetation on a bioprosthetic valve. This is a short axis view of the tricuspid valve, best obtained from proximal gastric location, with clockwise probe rotation at about 20–30°. The sewing ring of the prosthetic valve is clearly seen here and there is a mass attached to the leaflets indicative of vegetation.

362. **Answer: A.**

     Paradoxical embolism. The trans-esophageal echocardiogram image shows the interatrial septum with a large PFO in its typical location. The color flow shows left to right flow. This flow would reverse under situations of increased RA pressure such as straining, coughing and right heart failure. The orientation of the opening is favorable for thrombi originating in the inferior vena cava region to traverse the PFO to the left atrium even in the absence of raised RA pressure.

363. **Answer: C.**

     Fistulous communication between the aorta and the right ventricle. In addition to the fistulous communication, the image also shows aortic regurgitation. Fistulous communications generally result from rupture of an aortic root abscess. This may result in communications to the RA, RV, PA or the left ventricular outflow tract (LVOT). Other local complications include abscess of mitral aortic intervalvular fibrosa, leaflet aneurysm and perforation of the anterior mitral leaflet. One may also get an abscess in the ventricular septum, causing a ventricular septal defect after rupture.

364. **Answer: B.**

     Pulmonary valve endocarditis. This is a mid-esophageal image showing the aortic valve in short axis in the center and the RV inflow and outflow wrapped around it akin to the short axis of the aortic valve from a parasternal view. There is a large mass attached to the pulmonary valve consistent with vegetation. This is the likely source of his lung abscesses.

365. **Answer: A.**

     Coronary sinus. This is a low esophageal view partially cutting through the posterior A–V groove showing the coronary sinus.

366. **Answer: A.**

     Left atrial thrombus. This patient has a large left atrium with spontaneous echocontrast, with large masses originating form the left atrial appendage suggestive of thrombi. These masses were highly mobile and the patient had rheumatic mitral stenosis, though the mitral valve is not visualized here. Note that this patient is in sinus rhythm. In patients with mitral stenosis thrombi can form despite being in sinus rhythm because of stasis in a large atrium, another possible mechanism being paroxysmal atrial fibrillation. Myxoma generally arises form the atrial septum and mitral vegetations generally arise from the atrial side of the leaflets and generally do not grow to such a massive size.

367. **Answer: A.**

     Main pulmonary artery. This view is obtained from the mid-esophageal view, with anterior structures displayed away from the transducer and superior structures to the right. This is a typical tomographic view showing RVOT, pulmonary valve and main pulmonary artery. Part of the LVOT and aortic valve are seen posterior to this. Pulling the probe up slightly will show the distal PA and proximal branches can be seen from a much more proximal location in the esophagus from a horizontal plane.

368. **Answer: B.**

Stenosis. This is suggested by the increased transvalvular velocity associated with a slow deceleration time. The peak diastolic gradient is 16 mmHg, mean gradient is 8 mmHg and the pressure half-time is markedly prolonged at 250–300 ms, suggesting severe tricuspid stenosis. The pressure half-time method is not validated for calculating the effective orifice area of either native or prosthetic tricuspid valves. Generally a mean transvalvular gradient of >5 mmHg is suggestive of severe tricuspid stenosis.

369. **Answer: A.**

Thrombus. The differential diagnosis is between thrombus and left atrial myxoma. In this patient with a giant left atrium, who is likely to be in atrial fibrillation, this is more likely to be a thrombus. The fact that the mass in not pedunculated, and has a homogenous acoustic characteristic, favors a diagnosis of thrombus, though the possibility of myxoma cannot be excluded. If vascularity is shown in the mass by color flow imaging or contrast echocardiography with transpulmonary agents, then it would suggest myxoma. Lipomatous septum is dumbbell-shaped with sparing of the fossa ovalis. Lung carcinoma propagates to the left atrium through pulmonary veins and the mass generally originates in one of the pulmonary veins.

370. **Answer: A.**

Severe pulmonary hypertension Note that this is a systolic frame and the interventricular septum is flattened, indicating an RV pressure closer or equal to the LV pressure. The ventricular septum responds passively to the transmural pressure and hence generally is convex to RV both in systole and diastole because of the higher LV pressure. Severe TR with normal PA pressure would cause diastolic flattening of the septum, and the septum would be rounded in systole as the LV pressure is higher. In RV dysplasia, RV is dilated, thin walled with occasional aneurysms and the septum would be flattened in diastole. In RV infarct, PA pressure would be normal.

371. **Answer: A.**

Orthotropic heart transplantation. The ridge-like projection seen on the posterior left atrial wall is the site of anastomosis between donor and recipient left atria. The pulmonary venous side of the atria belongs to the recipient. The other anastomotic sites are the ascending aorta, superior and inferior vena cava and the pulmonary artery. Mitral annuloplasty ring will be seen posteriorly immediately superior to the base of the mitral leaflet and is rounded in cross-section. Classical maze or radiofrequency maze performed for atria fibrillation does not generally result in such ridge-like projections. The upper ventricular septum does not have a thin scooped-out appearance to suggest septal resection.

372. **Answer: C.**

Tricuspid valve prolapse. The density of the signal depends on the number of scatterers or the amount of regurgitant flow at the time the signal is generated. The increasing density of the signal from early to late systole suggests an increasing regurgitant volume through systole, which typically occurs in valve prolapse. In severe pulmonary hypertension, not only will the TR velocity be in the vicinity of 4 m/s but there is no differential signal density. Here the TR velocity reflects normal PA pressure. The flail valve causes severe TR from the very beginning of systole.

373. **Answer: A.**

Patent ductus arteriosus. This is the classic appearance of PDA with a communication between the distal arch and the origin of the left pulmonary artery. This view is helpful in diagnosing PDA as well as evaluating the morphology, length and diameter of the PDA, which are important for planning percutaneous PDA closure.

374. **Answer: A.**

Severe tricuspid stenosis. The diastolic velocity across the tricuspid valve is markedly increased with a very slow deceleration of the velocity profile. However the pressure half-time method is not validated for the tricuspid valve. The mean diastolic gradient across the valve at a mean heart rate of 47 beats per minute is 10 mmHg. A mean gradient of >5 mmHg is generally indicative of severe TS. The mean gradient is heart rate and flow dependent. The valve opening and closure clicks are suggestive of a mechanical prosthesis. TR velocity is systolic and Ebstein's anomaly causes TR rather than tricuspid stenosis. In tricuspid atresia, there is no flow across the tricuspid valve and RA emptying occurs through an atrial septal defect.

375. **Answer: D.**

Severe pulmonary hypertension with poor RV function. TR velocity is 4 m/s. This is consistent with an RA–RV gradient of 64 mmHg and PA systolic pressure of 80 mmHg in the absence of pulmonary stenosis. A very slow rise of TR velocity indicates a slow rise of RV pressure in early systole suggestive of RV dysfunction. The TR velocity profile lends itself to calculate RV dp/dt. In this patient the time taken for the TR velocity to rise from 1 to 3 m/s was 160 ms, corresponding to an RV dp/dt of 200 mmHg/s. RV dp/dt depends upon RV contractile function, PA pressure and LV contractile function. Normal RV dp/dt with normal PA pressure is 200–250 mmHg/s, but rises to 1000 mmHg/s in the presence of severe pulmonary hypertension associated with good RV contractile function.

376. **Answer: C.**

Severe. This is severe as judged by jet size, vena contract and proximal isovelocity surface area (PISA) radius. In addition the two-dimensional image shows lack of tricuspid leaflet coaptation, leading to wide-open TR. The mechanism is tricuspid annular dilatation and hence is functional, probably secondary to previous pulmonary hypertension due to mitral valve disease resulting in RV and RA dilatation, thus stretching the tricuspid annulus. This is repairable with tricuspid annuloplasty. Also note the partly seen mitral prosthesis. TR quantitations by using the three components of the jet are not well validated.

377. **Answer: C.**

Moderate or severe pulmonary hypertension. In patients with wide-open TR, the tricuspid valve may be fairly nonrestrictive, allowing RV and RA to behave virtually as a single chamber during systole. In such a situation the TR pressure gradient cannot reliably be calculated using the simplified Bernoulli equation as a considerable amount of energy may be expended in causing acceleration of the TR jet. In addition RA pressure may be very high, leading to underestimation of PA pressure. In this example, one can count the number of aliases to estimate the TR velocity at the vena contracta. There are four aliases corresponding to a velocity of 69×4, i.e. 2.76 cm/s. Though the pressure gradient is 30 mmHg, the patient is likely to have very high RA pressure, i.e. 20–30 mmHg, and because of wide-open TR the TR pressure gradient would have underestimated the pressure gradient. Hence the PA systolic pressure is at least moderate but more likely to be in the severe range in the absence of pulmonary stenosis. In such patients careful examination of the pulmonary regurgitant jet to get an estimate of PA diastolic pressure would be helpful.

378. **Answer: D.**

Replacement with a mechanical valve. This prosthesis probably is a bileaflet valve in view of the two areas of reverberations seen in the left atrium. A bioprosthetic valve would show struts in the periphery and thin leaflets in the center unless calcified. An annuloplasty ring is an echodense structure at the base of the mitral leaflet on the left atrial side with intact leaflets. This ring can be partial or complete. An alfieri stitch can be central or asymmetric and is simply a stitch that focally unites the tips of anterior and posterior leaflets and converts the mitral orifice into a double orifice, best seen in short axis view.

379. Answer. D. All of the above. Pre-intervention mitral flow is indicative of high left atrial pressure. This pattern is seen despite a heart rate of 92/min, as faster heart rates result in atrial predominance of ventricular filling. Postintervention mitral flow is suggestive of impaired left ventricular relaxation, which is consistent with normal or low mean left atrial pressure. Note that the heart rate is slower at 62/min. This patient had dilated cardiomyopathy with severe functional mitral regurgitation, which responded to diuresis and afterload reduction with a reduction of LV size and elimination of mitral regurgitation. Uncontrolled hypertension will reduce LV ejection performance, increase LV size and give rise to MR, as myopathic ventricles are exquisitely sensitive to afterload. As these patients have little or no functional reserve, anemia has a serious and deleterious effect on hemodynamics because of a reduction in oxygen-carrying capacity and a demand for higher cardiac output.

380. Answer. A. Thoracic aortic aneurysm. Thoracic aorta runs posterior to the left atrium, is rounded and on dynamic imaging is pulsatile. Turning the imaging plane by 90° would show the long axis of the descending aorta. The membrane of Cor triatriatum separates the pulmonary venous chamber from the lower part of the atrium and is best seen from parasternal long axis and apical views. The location is across the left atrium. Left pulmonary artery is not seen in the posterior mediastinum.

Chapter 20

381. The commonest location of this pathology is:

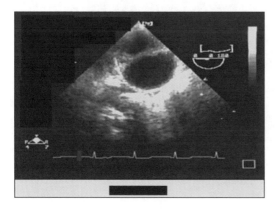

    A. Proximal ascending aorta
    B. Mid-aortic arch
    C. At the attachment of ligamentum arteriosum
    D. Junction of thoracic and abdominal aorta

382. This is a 27-year-old man with no prior medical history, presented with a three-month history of abdominal distension and lower extremity edema. Physical examination revealed severely elevated jugular venous pressure. He had normal left ventricular (LV) and right ventricular (RV) systolic functions. The most likely diagnosis is:

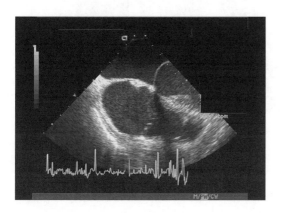

A. Superior mediastinum syndrome

B. Constrictive pericarditis

C. Restrictive cardiomyopathy

D. Cirrhosis of the liver

383. This patient presented with shortness of breath and cyanosis. The most likely cause is:

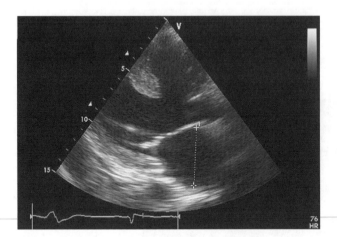

A. Ventricular septal defect (VSD) with Eisenmenger's

B. Atrial septal defect (ASD) with Eisenmenger's

C. Tetralogy of Fallot

D. Primary pulmonary hypertension

384. This pulmonary regurgitation (PR) signal is suggestive of:

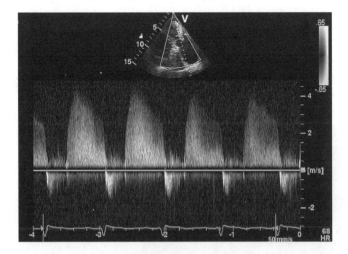

A. Severe pulmonary hypertension

B. Mild pulmonary hypertension

C. Normal pulmonary artery (PA) pressure

D. Severe pulmonic stenosis

385. The Doppler signals shown here are indicative of:

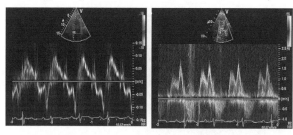

Doppler tissue imaging   Mitral inflow

   A. Normal LV diastolic function

   B. Abnormal LV relaxation with probable elevated left atrial (LA) pressure

   C. Abnormal LV relaxation with probably normal LA pressure

   D. Advanced restrictive cardiomyopathy

386. The continuous wave Doppler signal shown here is suggestive of:

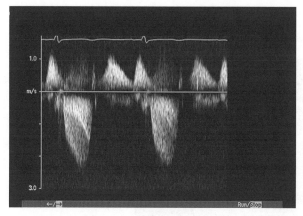

   A. Dynamic LV outflow obstruction due to systolic anterior motion (SAM)

   B. Critical valvular aortic stenosis (AS)

   C. Subvalvular AS due to a membrane

   D. Flow in and out of pseudoaneurysm

387. This signal was obtained from a right upper parasternal location with the patient turned to the right using a dedicated continuous wave Pedoff transducer. The likely diagnosis is:

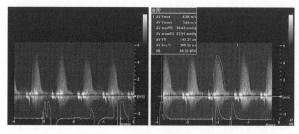

   A. Severe mitral regurgitation (MR)

   B. Severe tricuspid regurgitation (TR)

   C. Severe AS

   D. None of the above

388. The aortic valve shown in this image is:

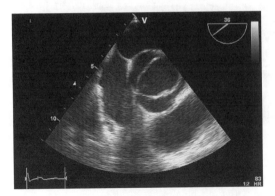

A. Unicuspid
B. Tricuspid
C. Bicuspid
D. Quadricuspid

389. What is the type of procedure that this patient has undergone?

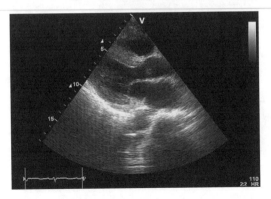

A. Mitral valve repair
B. Bioprosthetic valve aortic valve replacement
C. Orthotropic heart transplant
D. None of the above

390. This flow obtained from the distal aortic arch from the suprasternal notch is indicative of:

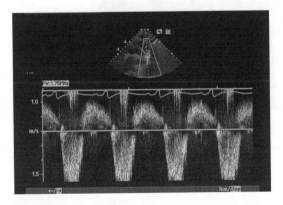

A. Severe AR

B. Aortic coarctation

C. Severe AS

D. None of the above

391. This image of the LV is indicative of:

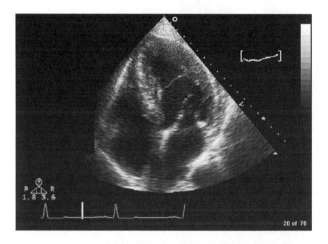

A. An LA thrombus

B. Left ventricular non-compaction

C. Bilobed LV

D. False tendon

392. Saline contrast echocardiography is suggestive of:

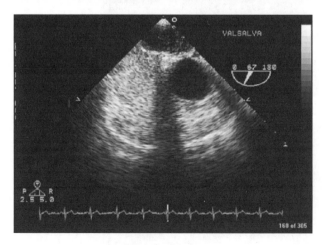

A. Patent foramen ovale (PFO)

B. Pulmonary AV fistula

C. Patent foramen or pulmonary A–V fistula

D. No right to left shunting

393. This trans–esophageal echocardiogram (TEE) image from the upper esophageal location shows:

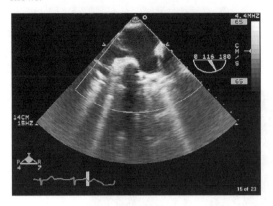

A. Left atrial appendage

B. Left upper and lower pulmonary veins

C. Left and right atria

D. Pulmonary artery branches

394. These two images obtained from the suprasternal notch are diagnostic of:

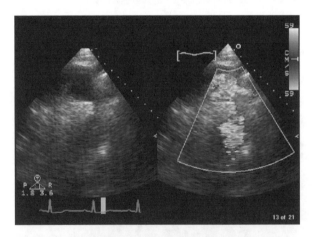

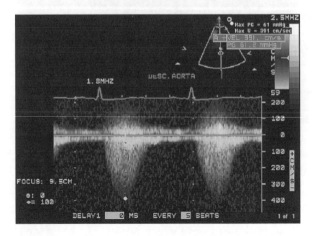

A. Coarctation of the aorta

B. Patent ductus arteriosus

C. Normal aortic flow

D. Pulmonary artery branch stenosis

(There is a full-colour version of the upper image in the plate section of this book)

395. This TEE image is indicative of:

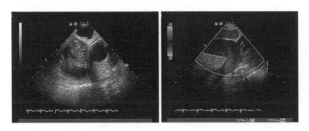

A. Left atrial myxoma

B. Right atrial myxoma

C. Lipomatous atrial septum

D. Vegetation of the tricuspid valve

396. What is the abnormality seen on this transthoracic echocardiogram?

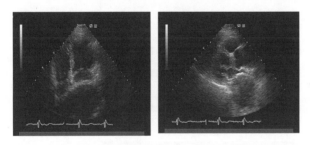

A. Aneurysmal left atrium

B. Partial absence of the pericardium

C. Thoracic aortic aneurysm

D. Loculated pleural effusion

397. The amount of MR in this patient is likely to be:

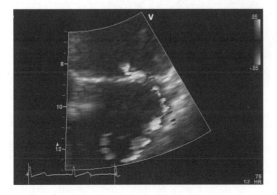

A. 1+

B. 2+

C. 3 or 4+

D. Cannot quantify

(There is a full-colour version of this image in the colour plate section of this book)

398. The cause of the systolic murmur in this patient is likely to be:

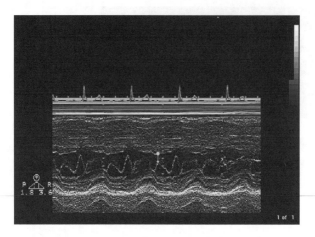

A. Rheumatic MR

B. Valvular AS

C. Hypertrophic obstructive cardiomyopathy (HOCM)

D. Aortic subvalvular membrane

399. This flow was obtained from the LV outflow tract from the apical view using pulse wave Doppler. This patient is most likely to have:

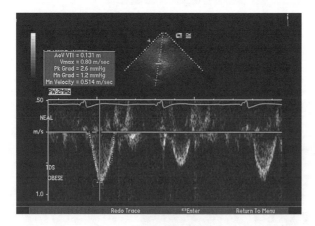

A. Severe congestive heart failure

B. Cardiac tamponade

C. Constrictive pericarditis

D. HOCM

400. This TEE image is indicative of:

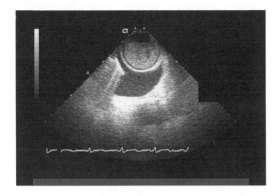

A. Left atrial thrombus
B. Aortic dissection
C. Saccular aneurysm of the aorta with a thrombus
D. Aortic pseudoaneurysm

Answers for chapter 20

381. **Answer: C.**

     At the attachment of the ligamentum arteriosum. This is a classic appearance of aortic transection with partial circumference disruption of the aortic wall. In a complete transection there will be discontinuity of aortic lumen and absent lower limb pulses. Transection generally is fatal with immediate exsanguinations into the mediastinum and the range of presentation includes discovery on TEE after a deceleration injury at one extreme to immediate death at the other extreme. The commonest location is at the junction of the arch and descending aorta where the ligamentum arteriosum is attached. Rarely, it occurs at the arch ascending aortic junction because of differential mobility of these three segments of the aorta and their attachments during rapid deceleration, as in a motor vehicle accident. In aortic dissection the intimal flap is thinner and the rounded shape of the aortic lumen is generally maintained. A mirror image artifact is on the far side of the aorta.

382. **Answer: B.**

     Constrictive pericarditis. This image shows marked pericardial thickening around the right atrium. On dynamic imaging, the right atrial wall was tethered to the pericardium along with classic signs of constriction, including septal bounce, respirophasic variations on transvalvular flows, preserved myocardial Em velocity and global pericardial thickening. His symptoms and physical signs resolved completely after pericardial stripping.

383. **Answer: A.**

     VSD with Eisenmenger's. There is a large VSD. Because of the size this is nonrestrictive and resulted in a large left to right shunt resulting in pulmonary hypertension. There is no overriding aorta here to suggest tetralogy of Fallot.

384. **Answer: A.**

     Severe pulmonary hypertension. The PR pressure profile reflects a PA to RV diastolic pressure gradient. Hence this patient's PA end systolic pressure is the square of early diastolic PR velocity + RV diastolic pressure, which would be similar to the RA pressure. In this patient this is calculated to be in the range of 80 mmHg, which would also be similar to the mean PA pressure. The PR end diastolic velocity is about 3m/s. Hence the PA diastolic pressure is 36 + RA pressure. This patient does not have significant pulmonary stenosis, as is shown by the accompanying systolic flow. In fact a markedly reduced duration is indicative of low cardiac output as well as a consequence of pulmonary hypertension.

385. **Answer: B.**

     An E' of <8 cm/s and an E/A ratio of <1 is indicative of abnormal LV relaxation. In addition mitral E/annular Em velocity ratio is 24. Normally this is in the range of 8–12. A ratio of >15 is generally indicative of high LA pressure. However this is applicable only in the absence of mitral stenosis. E-wave deceleration in this patient does not suggest mitral stenosis. The velocities were increased due to high cardiac output secondary to anemia. Advanced restrictive cardiomyopathy results in much higher E/A ratio and rapid E-wave deceleration (<150 ms).

386. **Answer: A.**

This late peaking ejection signal, which classically occurs due to dynamic left ventricular outflow tract (LVOT) obstruction due to SAM, occurs in HOCM. SAM is not specific for HOCM as it can occur in situations like postmitral valve repair, volume contracted states, hyperdynamic LV and severe mitral annulus calcification. Also note a lower velocity late peaking systolic signal inside the main signal. This is indicative of cavity obliteration and hence a hyperdynamic LV. Valvular AS and fixed subvalvular AS can result in a late peaking signal when they are severe or critical. A relatively low velocity signal in the presence of hyerdynamic LV and mitral flow suggestive of good LV filling are against this possibility.

387. **Answer: C.**

Severe aortic stenosis. This is a classic signal resulting from severe aortic stenosis with the flow directed towards the transducer. The timing of the signal is during ejection, as opposed to MR and TR signals that start earlier during systole, and also is less likely to pick up MR and TR signals from this location. This signal shown here is late peaking with a mean gradient of 53 mmHg indicative of severe or critical aortic stenosis.

388. **Answer: C.**

Bicuspid. This TEE image shows a bicuspid valve with anterior and posterior cusps. The anterior cusp is a conjoint one of right and left cusps. Two commissures can be seen and these should be traced to the annulus to count the number of cusps, as many bicuspid valves have partial commissural fusion only towards the annulus. In fact it has been shown in a pathology series that nearly 50% of so-called calcific AS cases are bicuspid. These patients may also have ascending aortic dilatation and there is association with coarctation of the aorta. Bicuspid aortic valve is common and occurs in 1–2% of the general population and needs endocarditis prophylaxis. Careful short axis evaluation of the aortic valve is mandatory for every patient referred for echocardiography.

389. **Answer: C.**

Orthotropic heart transplant. Please note a ridge-like structure in the posterior atrial wall, which represents atrial anastomosis between donor and recipient atria. Hence the left atrium is enlarged. Other areas of anastomosis include ascending aorta, main pulmonary artery and the vena cavae. Previously right atrial anastomosis was being performed, however this resulted in high incidence of severe TR due to tricuspid annular dilatation resulting from distorted right atrial anatomy.

390. **Answer: A.**

Severe aortic regurgitation. There is a prominent holodiastolic flow reversal indicative of a retrograde flow in the aorta indicating diastolic runoff of blood from the arch or the ascending aorta. The conditions that can cause this include significant AR, aorto-pulmonary window, ruptured sinus of Valsalva, fistulous communication to any of the cardiac chambers from the aorta and large coronary A–V fistula. Coarctation of the aorta may result in diastolic antegrade flow because of collaterals.

391. **Answer: D.**

This is a typical appearance of a false tendon running in the middle of the LV with no pathological significance. When such tendons are present in the apex they can be mistaken for thrombi and when these run along the anterior septum the thickness of the septum can be overestimated erroneously. This patient does not have significant LV trabeculation either in depth or extent to qualify for noncompaction. Though not all LV segments are shown, significant trabeculation denotes a noncompacted to compacted wall thickness ratio of 2.

392. **Answer: C.**

There are bubbles in the left atrium indicative of a right to left shunt. However, from a single frame the level of shunting cannot be determined. Hence the timing of appearance of bubbles in LA in relation to appearance in the RA is important. It is important to record at least 8–10 beats after the appearance of contrast in the RA. If the bubbles in the LA appear within 2–3 beats of its appearance in the RA the shunt probably is at the atrial level: if it appears later it is likely to be transpulmonary shunting due to pulmonary A–V fistulae. Examples of the latter include end stage liver disease and Rendu-Weber-Osler disease. In our laboratory we perform saline contrast echo without and with Valsalva's maneuver. The shunt in PFO is conditional to the transient rise in RA pressure and is produced by Valsalva, coughing and pressure over the abdomen. Movement of the atrial septum to the left ascertains a higher RA pressure. PFO diagnosis rate is higher by TEE and with lower limb contrast injection, as the direction of the PFO channel is directly in line with the inferior vena cava (IVC). Hence injection from the upper limb may be washed away by IVC flow and prevented from entering the PFO channel.

393. **Answer: B.**

Left upper and lower pulmonary veins. A tomographic plane a around 100–120° with the imaging plane superior and left of the appendage shows both left-sided pulmonary veins draining into the LA. Part of the image to the imager's right is cephalad and hence this is the left upper and the one on the right is the left lower pulmonary vein. Ability to get this image depends upon atrial size, pulmonary vein locations, relation of the pulmonary veins to the esophagus and body habitus, etc. but should be obtainable in over 90% of the patients. The LA appendage is a blind pouch.

394. **Answer: A.**

Coarctation of the aorta. This is a classical image of coarctation of the aorta. The two-dimensional image shows narrowing at the junction of the arch and descending aorta with turbulence on color flow imaging. The flow velocity across this narrowing was 3.9 m/s, indicative of a systolic gradient of 61 mmHg. This is indicative of severe coarctation. Other indicators of severity include a broader systolic signal, diastolic gradient and nonpulsatile flow in the descending aorta. Presence of arterial collaterals may reduce the gradient but the collateral-dependent flow in the descending aorta will be nonpulsatile.

395. **Answer: B.**

Right atrial myxoma. In this image there is clearly a right atrial mass, which is very large. Also note a very dilated IVC with no mass inside. The differential diagnosis includes myxoma, thrombus and metastatic tumor spreading through the IVC, such as renal cell carcinoma. The features that help to differentiate it are attachment of the mass (pedunculated attachment to the septum, likely to be myxoma), continuity of the mass in the IVC (renal cell carcinoma), presence of blood vessels in the mass on color flow (not a thrombus), presence of perfusion by transpulmonary contrast agents (thrombus has no enhancement, myxoma has mild enhancement, vascular tumors hyperenhance). This mass is too big for a valve vegetation.z

396. **Answer: C.**

Thoracic aortic aneurysm. The structure behind the left atrium is the thoracic aorta, which is normally seen in parasternal long axis view. The long axis of this part of the aorta can be visualized from the left parasternal view with the left parasagittal imaging plane.

397. **Answer: C.**

3 or 4+. This patient has a lateral wall-hugging jet reaching all the way to the roof of the left atrium. A wall-hugging jet area tends to be 40–50% smaller than a free jet area for a given regurgitant volume. In such patients examining the size of vena contracta, proximal isovelocity surface area (PISA) and calculating the effective regurgitant orifice area would be helpful for volumetric quantitation. Though the PISA is not well visualized in this patient, the diameter of the vena contracta is about 5 mm, which is consistent with at least 3+ mitral regurgitation. The mechanism of the lateral wall-hugging jet in this patient was a tethered posterior leaflet secondary to a rheumatic process. The other mechanism to cause a laterally directed jet would be a severely prolapsing anterior mitral leaflet.

398. **Answer: C.**

Hypertrophic obstructive cardiomyopathy. This is a typical M mode of systolic anterior motion of the mitral valve. The CD segment of the mitral valve (systolic segment) normally moves anteriorly during systole because of the translation of the LV and mitral valve anteriorly. However a CD segment slope greater than the slope of the posterior endocardium and the systolic mitral leaflet septal contact indicates SAM, which most commonly occurs in HOCM, but can occur in other situations too. The mitral valve opening is normal in this patient with a normal ejection fraction slope with thin leaflets ruling out rheumatic mitral stenosis. Fixed aortic stenosis due to a valvular or sub-valvular process does not give rise to any typical appearance of the mitral valve.

399. **Answer: A.**

Severe congestive heart failure. The beat in the middle is of lesser amplitude and duration, which gives a markedly lower time velocity integral compared to the beats on either side. A lower stroke volume and a weaker pulse with every other beat are called pulsus alternans and is suggestive of severe left ventricular systolic dysfunction. The change in amplitude is too rapid for respirophasic variation, which occurs in tamponade and constriction. Pulsus alternans is not seen in HOCM as it is mostly diastolic dysfunction and the LVOT velocity is higher because of SAM-related flow acceleration.

400. **Answer: B.**

Aortic dissection. This is a transverse section through the descending thoracic aorta. A smaller true lumen and a larger false lumen with a thrombus are seen. Also note fluid around the aorta indicative of left pleural effusion and this should raise the possibility of leaking aneurysm. In dissection or intramural hematoma, thrombus is inside the aortic wall and is covered by the endothelium, as in this case. In a saccular aneurysm with an intraluminal thrombus the endothelium is outside the thrombus. Pseudoaneurysm is characterized by an aneurysm bound only by adventitia outside the aortic lumen and communicating with the aorta through a narrow neck.

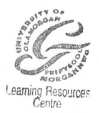